T0149539

BEHIND
THE SMILE

An inspirational journey
from disability to ability

Anja Christoffersen

BALBOA.
PRESS

A DIVISION OF HAY HOUSE

Balboa Press books may be ordered through booksellers or by contacting:

Balboa Press
A Division of Hay House
1663 Liberty Drive
Bloomington, IN 47403
www.balboapress.com.au
1 (877) 407-4847

Because of the dynamic nature of the Internet, any web addresses or links contained in this book may have changed since publication and may no longer be valid. The views expressed in this work are solely those of the author and do not necessarily reflect the views of the publisher, and the publisher hereby disclaims any responsibility for them.

The author of this book does not dispense medical advice or prescribe the use of any technique as a form of treatment for physical, emotional, or medical problems without the advice of a physician, either directly or indirectly. The intent of the author is only to offer information of a general nature to help you in your quest for emotional and spiritual well-being. In the event you use any of the information in this book for yourself, which is your constitutional right, the author and the publisher assume no responsibility for your actions.

Any people depicted in stock imagery provided by Getty Images are models, and such images are being used for illustrative purposes only.
Certain stock imagery © Getty Images.

Print information available on the last page.

ISBN: 978-1-5043-1461-9 (sc)
ISBN: 978-1-5043-1460-2 (e)

Balboa Press rev. date: 08/27/2018

Dedication

This book is dedicated to all the brave people who fight their battles in silence, seek acceptance, exhibit resilience, fearlessly express love, don't let anything hold them back and make it *despite* the odds.

Epigraph

"Nothing you can wear is more important
than your smile." - Connie Stevens

Foreword

Anja Christoffersen is a remarkable person, and this is a remarkable book.

The experiences related so thoughtfully in these pages tell her story with humour, wise reflection and an optimism that will be universally welcomed. This is neither a memoir nor an autobiography, but it is a revelation. Through anecdotes and vivacious interaction, the reader is taken on a journey from birth to early womanhood. There will be tears and belly laughs and above all admiration for a tenacious and resilient spirit.

I met Anja for the first time in a busy Melbourne coffee shop, in the company of her good friend and emerging writer, Greg Ryan and was dazzled by her confidence, maturity, intuition and quiet, worldly charm. I knew she had been born with an anorectal malformation of great complexity. I knew her life was in danger from her birth and I understood that the surgical efforts of many doctors had shaped the way in which she would live. Inspired by a determined mother Anja had turned her ominous prognosis on its head. Her effervescent laughter and sophisticated manner belied the physical difficulties that beset her now and for every other day of her life.

Several hours later I spent time at Melbourne's Royal Children's Hospital with Anja, Greg and the mothers of two other young girls who lived with similar congenital malformations to Anja's. The effect of Anja's presence was electric. It was profoundly moving to see both the mothers relaxing as they heard Anja relate her experiences. The anticipated difficulties of schools, work and relationships for the two younger girls almost disappeared in the laughter and joy of Anja's tales. The consequences of a life time of challenges seemed like minor obstacles in Anja's telling.

I have been fortunate since that day to spend time with Anja in a number of different social and educational environments and I now understand better the nuances of her life. She has talked about the joy of finding love that transcends the problems an alert world might expect. She declares with a passionate fire that she will not be defined by her illness. She undertakes activities, journeys and travails that most of us would and could not, but she knows that she will be prepared for inevitabilities in a way that is not required of others. All of this is captured in this erudite and charming book.

I recommend this chronicle unreservedly. It is uplifting, sensitive and irresistibly positive. It is also brave, and many of her readers will find the story challenging and disturbing. Anja like One in 5000 (a Foundation she has supported since its establishment) others across the planet knows that stories like hers need to be told so that adequate care, community support and dignity become the norm rather than the exception for those born with these malformations.

Anja, I know, trusts that her story thus far will give hope to others. She recognises that her future will look like her past. Daily physical disabilities will be encountered and resolved as far as possible. New obstacles will arise for her and the other 1 million families struggling to support their child through the inherent difficulties. The story will go on.

For now, this is a brilliant contribution to our hearts which will resonate with all readers and help motivate ongoing change in treatment, information and support for others with rare diseases. Enjoy and be inspired.

Les Cameron
Director of Film, Books, Anything P/L and the One in 5000 Foundation

Preface

At fifteen years of age I knew I had a valuable story that needed to be told. I committed to writing a book. I wanted to write about success, something I had not yet experienced in a typical sense.

Even so young, it had been years that the idea had been soaking into my head. When I fed someone a breadcrumb of insight into my life, they wanted the cake.

They weren't hungry for it before they got a taste and once they did, they wanted the recipe. How was I so happy, when I experienced so much suffering?

I was born into a game of chance. No blood test, scan, treatment or surgery could determine the odds for me. The dice was rolled often, and it would land favourably and unfavourably.

I was born with a congenital disability that deformed my digestive, skeletal, reproductive, circulatory, urinary and respiratory systems. Dressed fully you could not tell I was any different. It just teaches us not to judge a book by its cover.

I didn't realise my success was survival and experiencing it with a smile on my face. There was nothing more I had to accomplish in life than just be happy. Without happiness, the rest is meaningless – even our health.

So, what *is* behind the smile? Is it just a staged one to hide the truth or is it because I have learnt that no thought is important enough to harm me? No matter what our bodies are going through, it's all about how we *feel* emotionally, regardless of our circumstances.

Understanding that was my growth from the fifteen-year-old girl, studying in high school to be a doctor to a first-time author understanding that I can make a positive impact on the world. And all I had to do was show up with a smile and open heart, ready to share my story.

Acknowledgements

As it takes a village to raise a child, it takes strong women to love and nurture one of their own – two in particular. First, my mother, my inspiration, my rock, my hero and my blood. You have never failed to lift me up when I have fallen down and encourage me when I have lost hope. You keep me down to earth, grounded and ensure I don't grow an ego that is bigger than the size of my heart.

The second strong woman who has had a profound impact on my life is Alexandra – my godmother, my cheerleader, my "bullshit card" giver, my listening ear and my partner in crime. Thank you, Alex, for listening to my book three times, putting up with me writing until 4:30am and never failing to have a laugh with me.

I would like to thank my father, for everything he has done for me, and for always providing a shoulder for me to cry on when times get tough.

I would like to thank my agents David and Mary for believing in me and giving me the opportunity to follow my dreams.

I also want to pass sincere gratitude to those involved in the capturing of my book cover – Anthony Byron Photography, Emily Lane Makeup Artistry and Niki Teljega. Talent like yours cannot be matched.

I want to thank Peter, Jasmine, my beautiful friends and family for having my back, and still loving me even when I am living as a hermit writing, stuck in hospital or cancelling plans due to illness.

I want to extend a heartfelt thanks to Greg, Les and the ONE in 5000 Foundation for welcoming me with open arms and giving me a platform to connect with other people with my birth condition and their families.

Finally, I want to extend love to anyone and everyone who I have crossed paths with since my birth – family, medical staff, surgeons, friends, colleagues, teachers. You have all touched my life in some way and I wouldn't be the person I am without our interaction - no matter how small it was, even just a smile while crossing the street.

Introduction

Have you ever felt trapped, restricted, your true self enclosed, hidden in a box you have stamped with the label *'life'*? You cannot comprehend ever feeling like you have the freedom to be the author of your own story. When you are packing things away in the box, you put on the lid. If you are really worried about the box exploding open, you tape it shut to add extra resistance. Resistance to ensure when you explode out, you are not only ready, you are strong.

When you are the one in the box, you forget how it is packed. You forget there *is* a way out at all. The way out is never feeling undefeated, moping at the bottom and focusing on the walls closing in on you. To get out, you need to have a lot of strength and a lot of belief that you are more capable than you realise. You need to have belief that you *can* get out before the way will ever appear to you.

For those of you feeling as if there is no way out, then remember my next words. The only way out is up!

Burst out of the lid. Up with your thoughts to a place of positivity, and up so you can view the bigger picture objectively, and know the place that you are in. The success of the battle from a shifting of beliefs is the momentum that will take you even higher.

I

❦

Chance

Trust that what happens in your life is for a higher, positive purpose that you may be unaware of

A push on the middle of my back marked my cue. My legs felt like jelly perched on nail thin stilettoes. My heart raced as I took three large strides before seamlessly pivoting to face the length of catwalk. The audience were dark blurs in my peripheral. The shoes were high, the polished concrete smooth and slippery. The lights were blinding, and my skin was coated in a thick layer of goosebumps. I was overcome with a sense of achievement.

The blinding lights and goosebumps couldn't help but remind me of theatre. I felt a sense of familiarity. All eyes were on me. Rather than doctors huddled around examining me, the audience stayed in their seats as their eyes grazed up and down my body. The circumstances could not have been more juxtaposed. In this moment, I could not have felt more *alive*.

It is easy to allow your circumstances to become your identity. In this moment, there was no room for my 'alter-ego' - the 'disabled', weak girl - the personality I could easily slip into when I was spending my days in hospital or bed-bound. I left her back in Australia, she wasn't invited on this trip however she was definitely part of the journey to get there. Every visualisation since my 2015 New Year's Eve countdown centred around this moment.

I had no idea of the "how" of getting there, and that wasn't my focus. I trusted the details would take care of themselves. I knew the most important thing was to *believe* I could. Sounds stereotypical, I know.

Self-belief seems easy when things are going your way, but when life presents challenge after challenge, and obstacle after obstacle, giving up or dismissing a positive story is easy. There were many times I could have given up on myself. The doctors gave up on me ever living a "normal life" before I was even born. It would be celebrated if I could survive, let alone *live*.

When I became old enough to understand that my life wouldn't be "'normal'" I wasn't bothered by it. I didn't want a normal life, I wanted an extraordinary one. I made the decision that I would be happy despite my circumstances.

Once I understood that not everyone faced the same challenges that I would with my disability, I posed a question to myself; is being one in 10,000, or perhaps even one in 40,000 a blessing, or a curse?

It really is based on your perception. If you are the one in 30,000 that holds the winning lottery ticket, you're feeling blessed, but if you're the one in 465 that has had your ID stolen, you're feeling *very* frustrated.

To set the scene, it was 1981 and thick snow lined the streets of Denmark as the clear blue sky beamed from above. My Danish-born mother came from where she lived in Brisbane, Australia to hand-deliver gifts to her neighbour's brother. I've only mentioned two sentences and it's already obvious what happens.

Their first meeting was described with words like 'fireworks' when they retold the story. They tell me that when you meet the love of your life, you just know it. Mum, loving to create some controversial gossip in the small towns in Denmark decided to spend the next week at his place, as they just couldn't be without each other. Dad had been married previously and had a 7-year-old daughter and 17-year-old son, so despite such a passionate romance, unless mum could stay in Denmark, they couldn't be together.

The twist in the tale is *not* that mum found out she was expecting on her return home, but that she kissed him goodbye at the airport, and they fell out of touch.

In 1994, before telephone communication was properly utilised in love stories, my mum returned to Denmark to rekindle this love that nothing else was able to match. With the moral of the story being, 'you really should have called beforehand' she quickly found out that my father had gone to Australia for the wedding of his nephew. He was searching for her there! Luckily for fate, by the time my mother returned to Australia, my dad was still there. And just like that, as if thirteen precious years of their life had not passed, they picked up exactly where they left off.

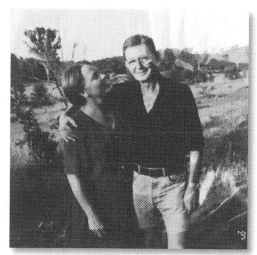

Mum and Dad

Even though they were oblivious to the set up, they were smart enough to not make the same mistake twice and, in that moment, realised they could not wait another 13 years, or even 13 days before being able to see each other again. They both got the logistics sorted out, Dad applied for Permanent Residency from Denmark based on his relationship with my mother and came to Australia to create a life together.

My parents decided to start a business together as mum's job required her to travel one third of the year and they didn't want to spend that time apart. Based on my mother's extensive experience in the education department, especially internationally, they decided on an International Education Consultancy business that facilitated International Students to study in Australia. They launched this in 1995 and recruited some staff. The success of the business skyrocketed.

My wild parents were enjoying home life as a DINK (Double Income No young Kids) couple, mum having assumed that she was too old to have children. Of course, I had another idea, and after a few hormonal changes in late 1997, Dad suggested she may be pregnant. In Aussie fashion, my 44-year-old Mum's five-star response was "Bullshit" but my 54-year-old father insisted otherwise and went to the chemist to get a test.

Funnily enough, my mother was in fact pregnant, three months along by this time.

Now that we have come to the stage where I have developed to be the size of a plum, my life had officially begun. For you to make your own judgement, on whether my rare condition is a blessing or a curse, you need to hear the full story, and here it is:

As the weeks flew by, my mother went in for the 28-week check-up with the midwife where she was measured from the top of her pubic bone to the top of her uterus, and it measured a lot larger than what you would expect for a woman at that duration. Concerned, the midwife arranged a scan straight away.

Mum went in for her ultrasound, and the technician started scanning, looking concerned and measuring things before excusing herself. She left the room and called for another technician until about four people had scanned Mum and were huddled around her. What flagged for them was they were unable to find the stomach in the scan.

Mum interrogated the technician, "If my baby doesn't have a stomach, can it survive?"

This scored a very timid reply of "no", almost inaudible. Mum's next question left everyone in the room silent, "So you are telling me that I will give birth to a baby, who will only be able to survive a maximum of a few days??"

They arranged a scan for my parents the following day with a special radiologist who would be able to find out more. Mum went home and researched "Foetus without stomach". This search produced very grim results. Many tears were shed that night.

Emotions were tense the morning of the specialist scan.

Mum went into the small ultrasound room at the hospital where the specialist scanned, identifying a cluster of abnormalities. In this scan, they uncovered:

V- VERTEBRAL: He could see there were vertebral abnormalities; scoliosis, hemivertebrae, extra lumbar vertebrae and missing bones in the sacrum.

A – ANAL ATRESIA: He could see the anus was imperforate.

C – CARDIAC: A hole in the heart was found.

TE - TRACHEOESOPHAGEAL FISTULA: He found that the food pipe was connected into the air pipe, going straight into my lungs. It was preventing fluid from getting into the stomach, and that was why the stomach could not be seen.

R – RENAL: He found there was only one kidney

L – LUMBAR: He was able to measure my limbs to ensure they were expected lengths, and thankfully they were.

Other abnormalities they could see from the scan included excess fluid in the amniotic sack and a single artery umbilical cord. Despite them finding out all these things about me, they were unable to tell my mother my gender.

Fortunately, the specialist radiographer had encountered this condition once before. He was confident to make the diagnosis from the 28-week scan.

The collection of medical defects was identified as a single birth disability "VACTERL Association". It was such a rare condition that there was no known cause or 101 guide on what it meant for the baby. There was a one in 10,000 to one in 40,000 occurrence rate. The survival rates were poor and there wasn't a story of hope anywhere to be found.

My parents were devastated and heartbroken. They were always perfectly healthy – no medical issues in the family.

Could the problem be a recessive gene rearing its head for the first time in family history? Could it be related to their age? Or some environmental factor? The doctors were unable to provide any reason, response or answer.

The medical team couldn't determine the extent of my issues until I was born. All they could do was monitor the pregnancy. The hospital began liaising with the surgical team in the children's hospital, just a maze of corridors away from where I would be born. They induced mum five days before my due date (Thursday) as the surgical team was on standby for Friday.

In a whirlwind of ultrasounds, blood pressure monitors and maternity clothes, the time flew by until it was the day mum was to be induced. I was due the following Tuesday. I was almost carried full-term which benefited me in terms strength, development and weight.

Funnily enough, if I was to be born on my correct birth date I would share it with Mums twin brothers.

Going into the hospital that morning in early July 1998, my parents were unsure if they would ever walk out of the hospital holding their baby. What they knew for certain was that they would not be able to leave the hospital the same people as they were when they arrived. The carefree nights cuddled up in front of the TV with a glass of wine were never going to be quite as carefree anymore.

Mum, heavily pregnant, waddled to the bed where she was to be induced twice. The first one appeared to have no effect, and after the second she was jolted into labour with contractions not too far about.

She was huge – carrying 7L of fluid, that when her water finally broke, it flooded the table and quickly overflowed.

With contractions so close together they assumed labour would be fast. Instead, from the morning, through the night, to the morning again, mum had fierce contractions. Dad had gone home to get some sleep as they both realised there was a very long night ahead of them.

As the doctors and nurses mutedly discussed what my plan was, a paediatric surgeon caught ear of it and joined the conversation. Quickly it was found that he was the perfect candidate to perform my surgery.

Dr B poked his head in to mum. By this stage it was the following morning and my delivery was closely looming. Dad was back after having a great sleep, much to the resentment of my exhausted mother.

"Could I take over your baby's care and surgery?" he questioned.

Mum and Dad wanted an expert. We were in a public hospital as they had no private health insurance and it was impossible for them to get any once they found out about my medical condition. Dr B had been training with a world famous Colorectal Surgeon overseas, who specialised in children with IA (Imperforate Anus) and Cloaca (only one opening). He had only returned from this training a mere month before my birth.

My life was to begin in this perfect synchronicity.

II

Survival

*And all anyone could take comfort in, was that this time
too shall pass*

In the final hour of a 26-hour labour, mum was unable to dilate past a
certain point and my vitals began dropping fast. They rushed mum to
theatre for an emergency caesarean. As soon as I was pulled from mum's
tummy, the focus was on me - my parent's new daughter (despite their
'intuition' saying I would be a boy)! They removed mum's epidural and she
experienced immediate drug withdrawals, beginning to shake.

I was ripped from the womb, placed on my mother's breast for
seconds while she convulsed, unable to touch me – nowhere near long
enough to bring my mother's breast milk down. There was no time to
spare. The eagle eyed medical team quickly whisked me away, preparing
me for surgery.

I was put in an incubator as the surgeons cleared an operating theatre.
I was hooked up to machines in minutes. The nurses insisted on taking
a polaroid photo so my parents "had a memory of me" if I were to die in
surgery. These were the times where film took days to weeks to develop,
and an instant photo was confirmation that every second was of great
value.

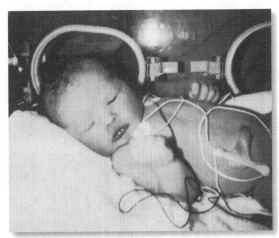

My Polaroid at Birth

It was made clear to my grief-stricken parents that I may not live through my first surgery. It was a life or death situation.

I was wheeled across to the children's hospital, for my first surgery at five hours old. My father followed behind the trolley and sat outside the operating theatre alone, waiting for an update so he could walk across and let my mother know. Mum had her baby ripped away from her and was now in the position of listening to other mothers cooing about their healthy, gurgling newborns. She felt like a failure as she couldn't have a natural birth, or a healthy baby – a feeling no one should ever have to experience.

Mum was told to try and begin pumping as breastmilk would be very healing for my little body once I was out of surgery. This was a huge struggle as the lack of contact with me made it almost impossible for her body to have the hormonal change needed for breastmilk to come down.

With this added pressure, mum was not having much luck. She sat next to these other mothers, from different cultures, third-world-countries, young and old, educated and uneducated, and she just could not come to terms with why her baby had all these issues with her body. She had always done everything right with her life – she had stable grounding, multiple university degrees and owned her own home, but she could not even produce milk or a healthy baby.

About two hours into the surgery, the surgeons came out and informed Dad that I had a 'high confluence' cloaca with a long cloacal channel, where my intestine (no rectum), bladder/urethra and two vaginas were joined together high up in my body, leaving one main opening. This flagged a lot of concerns, the least of them being my duplicated reproductive organs. The confirmation of bowel incontinence was made, as well as the strong probability of urine incontinence as well.

When my parents heard this, they could not help but cry. They had fears for their child's physical wellbeing as well as my emotional wellbeing – bullying, being the 'smelly kid' and being an outcast throughout my life.

As the cloaca was not functional and was impossible to leave as is, they gave me a vesicostomy (bladder) and colostomy (bowel).

The other issue that needed an immediate fix, was the tracheal-oesophageal fistula (joining of my food pipe and air pipe). They operated; making an incision under my arm to remove a rib and access the deformity. My food pipe was not even formed, having no connection with my stomach (oesophageal atresia). This pouch was joined up to my air pipe, causing anything I would swallow, including saliva, to flow back into my lungs.

At just over 10 hours old, I was wheeled out of theatre up to the Neonatal Intensive Care Unit (NICU) for close monitoring and recovery. With medical assistance I could now eat, breathe, poo and pee thanks to the brilliance of the surgeons. As I had just had surgery on my food pipe and bowel, I was fed through a Nasal Gastric Tube and fluids through an IV to avoid anything touching the fresh surgical wounds. I was also on oxygen to help me to breathe.

My parents had to fight to see me in NICU as I was in a critical condition. I could not be picked up or even bathed as I was so weak. Mum was only able to come for short periods of time in a wheelchair from the Women's hospital where they were caring for her post-caesarean.

The surgery was deemed a success, but there was still no greater guarantee of survival at this time.

By day three, I was still not out of the woods and Mum discharged herself from hospital. The crash of hormones was in full swing and combine that with a baby who was barely surviving, my usually joyous mother was slipping into a post-natal depression that she did not admit to anyone.

By day four, the 14th of July, my parents had their "first cuddle" with me, also captured by the dreaded polaroid camera that depicted I most certainly was not on the home stretch just yet. Whenever my fragile body was touched the medical alarms would begin blaring, worrying my parents.

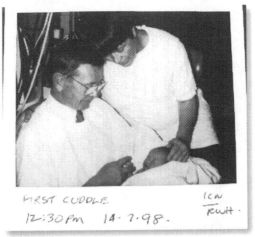

FIRST CUDDLE
12:30 Pm   14·7·98·
ICN
RWH·

Mum and Dad's first cuddle (Polaroid)

At five days old I pulled out the nasal-gastric tube through my nose from the pit of my stomach, with my free hand. Clearly, I had decided that this NGT tube was uncomfortable and unnecessary. The doctors didn't have the same idea as I did, and unfortunately it was put back in as quickly as I had taken it out.

I remained in the Intensive Care Unit for a week, before being put into a special care ward for a further three weeks. The STOMA nurses gently guided my mother on how to manage my care needs with the colostomy and vesicostomy.

Even though it had only been a month, issues were already arising with the colostomy. The contact of the bag on my wafer-thin skin was enough to make it bleed. It became so raw the bag would rarely stick.

The vesicostomy was reasonably easy to manage. It was a low cut to expose the bladder to the outside, so the urine could get out of the body. The advantage of such a low cut, meant that it could be covered by nappies and seem relatively "normal".

My birth came at a perfect time for my parents if there ever was one. Their company was established (3 years old) and they were their own bosses, so could manage and amend their own working hours to care for me. The business was still booming with the help of their staff.

I was released from the hospital at one month of age. I had white blonde hair, blue eyes and could drink breastmilk from a bottle as I still wouldn't latch.

It was hard for my parents as they did not feel like they could celebrate my birth like a typical couple and family could. They were unsure of how

I would cope in the future, the length of my life expectancy and if I would be able to survive through the rollercoaster with my health that was soon to follow.

When I was born there was a cluster of about 5 VACTERL babies with slight variations, from Brisbane that we knew of. To be diagnosed with this condition you must have at least three associated defects, and I was quite over-qualified.

Mum kept in contact with these other mothers of VACTERL babies and had found a specialist that described these clusters occurred in little old Brisbane every three to five years at that time. It was extraordinary how many similarities, as well as differences there were between us, especially in our varied experiences.

In this circle of VACTERL mums, they could each gain knowledge and perspective off each other, and not feel quite so alone.

One of the wise things they were able to teach each other was to puncture the colostomy bag to let gas escape. Mum discovered this after having my colostomy blow off in public, spraying poo everywhere and making a large bang.

Despite wearing a colostomy bag and having an open incision for my bladder to empty, my joy and zest for life wasn't dampened. Mum would take me with her to work meetings and even to the beach or public pools. I would wear sweet frilly pink swimmers and "swim" through the water in my parents' arms. My parents always called me a water baby - joking that there was so much fluid in mum's pregnant belly I was always swimming laps during the pregnancy, kicking off her lungs, stomach or bladder! This meant once I was born, they quickly found I felt comfortable in water so would take me swimming often.

I had a great babyhood with my parents. Despite bouncing in and out of hospital with a weakened immune system, I had a vibrant lifestyle. I was delayed with my physical development however no one seemed concerned given my surgeries.

I never crawled as a baby. I tried a few times and found the colostomy bag would dig in and disintegrate my paper-like skin, leaving me with a bag full of blood. There have been studies that show a key development stage of a child is when crawling as it helps them to develop good coordination. I can safely say the studies were right, and I was not destined to be an athlete.

Once the immediate issues were resolved, I underwent further testing to check that the hole in my heart had fully resolved and was functioning normally. The doctors diagnosed me with bradycardia, which is a fancy word for a slow heart rate. It wouldn't be a problem by itself, however it meant on occasion the amount of oxygen being pumped through my body wasn't enough. This further enhanced my respiratory impediment.

Due to how I developed (or didn't) in the womb, the walls of my air pipe and bronchioles were weak. This was confirmed by further medical imaging and scopes under GA, as it hadn't strengthened on its own as I had grown. I was diagnosed with Primary Trachaeobronchomalacia where the cartilage and muscles are not strong enough in that area to hold your airway open due to surgical intervention. In my case, my air pipe had collapsed into a figure 8.

I would struggle to suck in enough air and could not breath lying flat down. At this stage, I was too young to begin breathing physiotherapy to build the muscles. The doctors hoped that the muscles would strengthen as I grew. In the interim, it meant a raspy TOF 50-years-pack-a-day-smoker's cough and a low oxygen saturation.

My mum has many memories of taking me out to restaurants, grocery shopping and the like, and getting horrible looks when I started to cough. It is a nasty "TOF cough", triggered by as little as an itch in the back of my throat. This cough sounds like I died of pneumonia *yesterday*. When I would cough in public people criticised my mum for not keeping me at home or taking me to the hospital as it sounded so severe.

With the TOF repair, I experienced severe gastro-oesophageal relax (GOR). Laying down I could not breathe, and on occasion the reflux would aspirate into my lungs, deteriorating my respiratory system further. At times I would spit and vomit up blood, until I was put on reflux medication 'for life'. Mum would sit up throughout the night with me in her arms, so I could breathe and not be in reflux pain.

At six months I moved directly from a dairy diet to finger foods. Mum had tried with baby puree however any sloppy food would get stuck in my throat like mucus and I would cough, splutter and choke. Where the muscles were cut in the reconstruction, the natural swallowing contractions of the upper section of my food pipe did not 'communicate' with the lower part. I would have to wash all my food down with water and often cough and vomit to try and expel things that got stuck.

Being on solids I was growing well. The surgeons decided to embark on my reconstructive surgery as they believed I was strong enough by this time.

The surgery date was booked as my parents' anxiety soared. The first six months was a montage of challenges, with every night being another time where my mother had to stay up, keeping my body at an angle where my reflux would be minimised. Every meal was a chance of choking where I would need to be fed and monitored closely and each day my skin disintegrated more from the colostomy.

Would this surgery, despite it being necessary, create problems with my bowels, bladder and reproductive system? Would I come out of it with more issues than I had going in? Would I even wake up from the surgery?

The answers to these questions were not definitive.

III

—⁂—

Theatre

You are never given a challenge that you are not strong enough to overcome

My parents signed the consent form acknowledging the high risk of the surgery. As the pen was handed back to the doctor, I was wheeled into theatre.

The malformation I had – cloaca - is one of the rarest and complex abnormalities, and a challenge to reconstruct. Think about it for a moment, two vaginas, bladder and intestine all as one opening. I would not even know where to begin (that's why I am not a surgeon)!

There are so many doctors around the world that are unfamiliar with this condition, and a lot of those who are 'familiar' have only heard or read about it. It is rare to find a doctor who has experience with it. Thankfully my surgeon *was* an expert. Even my terrified parents felt confident in my surgeon's ability.

I went in to the operating room around midday on the 11th of January 1999 for my 'Pull Through' also known as PSARP (Posterior sagittal anorectoplasty) surgery.

In one confident sweep, I was cut the whole way from my clitoris to the back of my bottom forming the butt cheeks as well as an incision on my abdomen. This opened me up, allowing the reconstruction to begin.

They pulled my intestine to the outside forming the anal opening. There was no rectum, sphincter, nerves or natural muscles surrounding it, meaning in my case, regardless of the success I would *always* be incontinent.

My urethra was tucked up near my clitoris as it has been found that urinary continence is best with this placement. As there was no extended tube for the urethra or vagina to reach the outside of my body, they had to construct this with tissue from the small bowel. This is a very effective method however means that I do not have the natural bacterial make-up to provide resistance against urinary tract infections (UTI) and pelvic inflammatory disease (PID).

In my reproductive reconstruction, they had to join the two vaginas into one opening leaving the two separate uteri, with a single ovary off each, both there.

Those three and a half hours in theatre felt like an eternity to my concerned parents. I came out of surgery weak and in horrible pain. My medical records reflect that no amount of IV morphine was able to give me relief that evening or throughout the night. My mother was very teary, completely overwhelmed by the whole situation.

She stayed with me in the hospital, sleeping very carefully beside me in my hospital cot.

After a long, painful night, with the nurses taking observations every 2 hours, I woke up alert and appearing to be much happier. My nose, easily irritated, was raw from scratching it from the morphine, but I was having a good time being pain free! Despite my improved condition, I had to remain in hospital for a further week and stay as still as possible to allow things to heal.

They sent a geneticist to see my parents that morning and the geneticist said to mum that she should not have to worry about having any more children with this condition as it is highly unlikely that she would get another VACTERL kid. My mother asked if they knew what caused VACTERL and they said no. Mum proceeded to ask how the geneticist could say that with such certainty.

It was clear that the cause was a mystery to everybody.

By February, three weeks after my pull through surgery, I was admitted to hospital again to go under anaesthetic to have my stitches removed, a urethroscopy and my first anal dilatation. After this procedure I stayed in hospital overnight and in the morning the STOMA nurse came to teach my mother how to perform anal dilatation on me.

As I had been operated on, it meant the opening would heal back to a small size made inflexible by rigid scar tissue. Anal dilatation had to begin before the scar tissue formed. This involved using hard plastic rods to force into my bottom to break open the skin causing it to bleed. The aim was that it would grow back bigger each time as each rod size increased.

My mother understood it was a necessary daily procedure to have a functional anus. Despite my screams and tears, she pushed through with the treatment.

For the next 6-12 months I needed to have anal dilatation every day.

My mother had never even put in my head that doing the anal dilatations was horrible or would be traumatic for me. I admired mum for being strong enough to endure it. I never had any negative associations with dilatations apart from the temporary pain. I can understand that I am better off in the present day because of it however am surprised there haven't been any other methods developed.

By mid-March, just under 6 weeks after my previous surgery and vigorous anal dilatation under sedation, I went under general anaesthetic again for another forceful anal dilatation and cystoscopy to monitor a vesico-vaginal fistula they had found post pull-through surgery. This went off without a hitch and I was able to progress to the dilator the next size up after that procedure, coming out with my anus bruised and bleeding.

Once all my wounds had healed there came the time to close the colostomy and vesicostomy that were done in procedures ranging from 40 minutes to two hours in length, one month apart.

I could now pee, poo and have potential to function sexually. My parents understood that I wasn't "fixed" however were grateful that the worst was now over.

Steering clear of the operating theatre, we began to explore my new life - how my bowel was going to function and if it would be as simple as we had hoped.

I was into nappies like any 8-month-old baby and *finally* had my first dirty nappy. This was celebrated by my parents and surgeons. You can tell we really value the small things in life - a benefit of perspective when there is an unwell person in the family.

I started on a strict laxative program as my body did not have the natural contractions in the bowel to push the poo through my body.

With every dirty nappy, I got instant nappy rash as my bottom hadn't built up the tolerance of having anything on it. Especially with my solid diet, the acidity would corrode the skin until I had nappies filled with blood. It would only take 20 minutes or less before beginning to bleed.

I would always need immediate changes where possible, however this was a challenge. I didn't have any bowel control so as the poo went through my intestine it would just keep coming out and could even result in it being a constant flow. No matter how closely monitored there would always be a dirty nappy left on too long. I was only able to get relief once mum found a perfect cream to soothe and heal the area.

The laxatives increased my bowel flow meaning it was inevitable for faeces to contaminate my vagina and urethra.

After 4-5 hospital admissions for UTIs within the six months following my pull through and ostomy closures I was put on prophylactic antibiotics to try and keep me well, and my solitary kidney safe. I had no nerves to detect stinging when I peed, so I could be asymptomatic until it went into my kidney.

As antibiotics deteriorate good bacteria in the gut, I was also on acidophilus to restore my body. If I missed a tablet I would end up with a raging thrush infection. It was a very careful balance to keep me in good health at this stage.

As the doctors began looking ahead at my future, it was clear that there was a need for social continence, as I was not given the luxury of wearing diapers for life. How this was arranged, was in a bowel management regime, and we were offered two options.

One; what they called a "plug" where they create a little hole into the intestine where you can inject a formula and wash out all the bowel underneath that area. My sweet mother argued against this as she suspected I would want to run around in a bikini on the beach without having to worry about it.

I chose the second option - enemas or "bowel washouts", nicknamed WOs. Mum would use a long catheter, putting it 10-15cm into my bottom and injecting a 60mL solution (glycerol/saline) to irritate the bowel in an attempt to empty it. I would have to lay on my side, curled up in a foetal position before jumping up, holding the bluey to my bottom as the mixture would begin running out immediately. I would then sit straight on the toilet/potty. This process would take around one hour, and after that I would usually have 2 hours where 'leakage' would continue. I began this at 1 year of age.

When I began having WOs, my body was ultra-sensitive. For approximately one year, with every WO I would be covered in goosebumps, vomiting, shaking, dizzy and very unwell. It was effective in keeping me clean most of the time, so we decided to just push through with this treatment. I always assumed in my teen years that I would train my muscles to develop bowel function and control so I could live without doing enemas.

Even with WOs and laxatives, due to how my body operated I faced the fate of chronic constipation.

When I started to block up, immediate action was needed. There were many occasions where I could not even keep water down. My mother would take me to hospital and tell the doctors that I was constipated, for them to look at my relatively flat stomach and dispute it. Of course, after abdominal X-Rays each time, it was confirmed that I was very blocked. I would be given an adjusted program of laxatives and bear the consequences of the impending UTI from my lack of bowel control.

I had made it through so many challenges, and it looked like I was going to survive the wrath of my birth condition. After I passed my first birthday, my parents were confident enough in my health to hold a christening.

My sister and her partner flew over from Denmark for the occasion set on the 8th of August. This was such a special day for everyone in my family, as it signified being out of limbo-land with my health, and was a sign that I was here to stay.

All my family gathered at a beautiful Lutheran church in Brisbane City, as Danes are traditionally protestant, and some of my cousins had been confirmed in that same church. The family filed in through the open doors, everyone seeming to wear black, as if it was my funeral. Perhaps it signified the funeral of my old self – the baby that was constantly ill and in hospital, and it would be the rebirth of my healthy, vibrant self.

Soon after these celebrations, as I had cut back on laxatives to reduce the chance of UTIs from infrequent changes, I got blocked up. I was vomiting up my own poo and couldn't even keep a cup of water down as I was so full up. I was admitted to hospital and had 'Go Lightly' pumped into my stomach through an NGT tube – placed in under general anaesthetic for my bowel obstruction at 17 months old. For five days straight, we all waited before I had a single bowel motion. The food ladies, cleaners, and everyone on the ward was patiently waiting, and cheering once something happened!

I was obviously coming of age where I had to be toilet trained. This is challenge enough for any mother, let alone one with a child who couldn't even feel when they needed to poo!

As I had begun having the washouts, I would always be on the toilet straight after them, so that was easy. For peeing and other pooing from the laxatives, mum bought me this mint green potty chair, with a nice backing for me to lean on, and a table that went around my waist. Now *this* was awesome.

I would sit on the front deck of our house naked on the potty with some nice finger food on the table in front of me. I was very content as I watched dad mow the lawn, and mum trim the hedges.

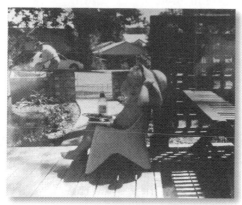

Chilling on the potty

Quickly, I learnt that if I needed to pee and poo, I just needed to go to the potty. Mum describes it now as quite an easy experience – but who knows if she is bluffing!

As my finger foods became more diverse, my choking incidences became more frequent.

To make the Guinness Book of World Records for the most random surgeries, I had to be anaesthetised for the doctors to remove first a blueberry (at 16 months), and then into surgery again five months later to remove a 'large grape' (at 21 months) from my oesophagus as it became lodged above the aortic arch!

SOMEHOW, I made it to two years of age, and through at least 8 surgeries. There may have been more, but I am not planning on "reading" doctors handwriting and going through 2,000+ pages of medical records.

Mum was very aware that I would have issues physically for life. Being a teacher, she began a little 'education' rampage, insisting that I would at least be smart.

As my parents worked so closely with universities, and I spent a lot of time in and out of the office even as a baby, instead of having cute animals or drawings or mystical creatures on the "roof" of my pram, to lay and look up at, I had postcards of the different universities in Queensland.

Mum would read books to me every night before bed. Books were my favourite thing at the time and I would follow along the words mum was reading. I would also have the freedom to draw and try to write and was able to write my own name perfectly by the age of two and a half.

Dad, of course, wanting to add his own educational flare, would teach me about some cars and motorbikes, and hearing the different engine sounds to identify them when I couldn't even see them.

My parents have a video of me at the age of two, standing on top of an outdoor table in the breezeway between sections of our house, and I hear the postman come on his bike.

Dad was filming me, and he asked me "who is that Anja?" to try and get me to say, "it's the postman" and everyone watching the video to think I was so clever. Instead, little sass-pot Anja said with a smartass undertone, "Well it is definitely *not* a Harley." From then on, I had won my dad's complete adoration.

My parents had not made me aware that I was any different to other kids or wrapped me in cotton wool. I knew I had a condition called VACTERL and had some special friends that would go to the hospital a lot like I would. Apart from that, you couldn't tell. When I was well I acted like any other happy-go-lucky child.

As my health had been stable, I had my first trip back to Denmark for my sister's wedding. I loved seeing my sister and family again, as well as exploring Denmark – my parents' homeland.

I spent some time at the summer house overlooking the beach. These women and men would arrive and begin taking off all their clothing, leaving it on the sand and strolling the whole beach stark naked. After their dip they would stroll back to where they left their clothes, not to put them on but to lay there and sunbake naked.

As I would look at all these Danes on the beach, young and old, slim and curvy, I thought it was fascinating how no two bodies are the same. I knew that some people had dimples in their thighs, others had ribs showing, and some had marks on their skin. I could understand that everyone was different, and I knew I was too, especially with my scars.

Growing up with this mentality and awareness was able to really help me accept and love my body, but of course at this stage I was too young to know any different.

Breathing in cool European "Summer" air, my chest began cracking and illness began to flare again...

IV

Admissions

Trust that even the worst of times occur to instigate positive change

40-degree temperatures were common for me, sometimes even higher. In and out of hospital, the doctors always used latex gloves, until at a young age I had experienced such overexposure to them, that I developed an allergy. Because I was in hospital so often, my veins had also collapsed due to the amount of cannulas and blood tests I had previously. I had to have cannulas put in my feet and legs often, and even in my neck when all other veins had collapsed.

Between 10:00pm and 3:00am were the magical hours of the night where I would wake up in the car on the way to hospital. My breathing would be so laboured, crackly and raspy that my mother would be scared that I would drown in my own mucus. I would be coughing so violently that my whole ribcage would feel bruised. I remember to this day the long nights dotted through each year where I would be coughing non-stop overnight and exhaust every option of heat rub and cough lolly possible.

Pneumonia was so common for me that everyone in my family could diagnose it straight away, as well as any medical professional could, just from watching my symptoms every 1-3 months. My mother should have been given her PhD in respiratory illnesses by this stage.

Surrounding my second birthday, I went into hospital three times, each time backed up with a history of pneumonia, an oxygen saturation of 85-90% and a letter from my GP. They took me in for a day, or even just hours in emergency and sent me home with antibiotics. Each time it was getting significantly worse, and mum, risking seeming like a psycho-overprotective mother, took me back time and time again.

Within 24 hours of my second discharge, my condition worsened. My mother was persistent enough to take me into the hospital as she was too scared to manage my condition at home. She could see the skin in between my ribs been sucked in with every breath I took and nostrils flaring. Once arriving at the hospital, they gave me Ventolin as they were trying to do anything to help me. My breathing was so horrible that they couldn't believe that it was *just* pneumonia and thought I must have some sort of Asthma as well.

After having the Ventolin, my heart rate sky rocketed. I was sitting up as I could not breathe lying down and started crying complaining of shooting pain going down my left arm. Suddenly, my body slumped back, heart stopped, alarms set off and my mother was pushed out of the room as a medical team came in for resuscitation. They managed to revive me and moved me to ICU to be monitored for 24 hours, before being sent to the ward.

It took this incident for my recurrent pneumonia to be taken seriously. I can give doctors so much praise – I would not be alive without them, but I can also give them so much criticism, as sometimes they *do* miss things. I was on IV antibiotics and litres of oxygen each day. Finally, about a week later, I was able to be discharged after the pneumonia FINALLY subsided. This was my 25th episode of pneumonia.

This was when we had to get something done. I was getting pneumonia so frequently and was being admitted to hospital with it more regularly than one could imagine. My respiratory specialist recommended doing a "Spring Clean" - where they put me under GA and 'vacuumed' out my lungs. My doctor said that during this, they were finally able to remove a mucus plug in the lower left lobe, that was majorly responsible for the recurrent pneumonia. When taking out the plug, she was able to take two steps back from the table, with this thick plug still stringing together from her to the pit of my lungs.

Once I had this procedure my pneumonia cleared up significantly, and I began to only get it 2-3 times a year rather than every month or so.

I started on breathing physiotherapy for an hour daily to strengthen my lungs and develop muscles to hold my air pipe open independently.

Each breathing exercise would drain and exhaust me, as my air pipe was so collapsed that I couldn't suck in or blow out enough air.

My hospital visits continuing to be frequent, I became besties with the nurses in the Ward I would frequently stay in. I spent my third birthday in hospital and as a surprise, my favourite nurse made and brought in a moist chocolate cake for my birthday that she had made herself! It was dairy free, especially for me.

The other great thing about my birthday is that it falls around a similar time to when the Royal Exhibition in Brisbane – the EKKA is on. The EKKA is the best thing ever for a kid, and even some adults. There are rides, showbags, animals, carnival food, shows and fireworks. Instead of being there, I was wound up in hospital, looking out the window watching people walk to the showgrounds only 100 metres away.

My mother, being the best mum of all time, discussed with the nurses and they decided to let me unplug my drip for an hour while mum took me in a wheelchair, with a mask on, over to the EKKA to see the 7pm fireworks. I was SO EXCITED.

I wore warm pyjamas and a blanket and was wheeled to the main entrance by mum. They thought I was so cute, and as there was only an hour left, they let us in for free. Mum wheeled me through the bright colourful lights of the rides, sideshow alley with all the carnival games to the stadium where the fireworks were going to be.

We watched the firework show and it was spectacular. I was so incredibly happy and knew two things in that moment as a three-year-old. First – my mother had my back, no matter what. Second – Even when I was feeling sick, I could still be excruciatingly, amazingly happy.

Three-year-old Anja made some great "new age resolutions" and decided to start ballet. I loved ballet and the thought of being beautiful, graceful and centre stage. On Saturday mornings I would go to classes with my two best friends from day care.

Along with ballet, I decided to start beading necklaces in my free time. I got some beads and started.

I had always been a child of experience and fascinated by the human body as I knew that my similar-aged cousins' bodies did not work the same as mine did.

I decided to do some research of my own and wanted to find out what it was like for there to be a bead in my nose. I knew some people had nose piercings, so putting a bead inside my nose could be a new trend.

I shoved one of the larger beads up there. It didn't feel so bad, and I had put it in the right way, so I would still be able to breathe through the hole in the bead. So, the bead was in my nose and I thought that was cool. I put in my tiny fingers to try and scrape it out, but it only pushed it in further.

Really relaxed, and not alarmed at all, I recruited my horrified mum to try and help me get it out. I tried blowing my nose, pushing it down from the outside, carefully using a chopstick – nothing would work! Off to the hospital I went, not very impressed with having to get a scary doctor in a big white coat to dig it out for me.

At the hospital, they were trying to get it out, but they couldn't! So, I had to go in for another surgery... removing a plastic bead from my nose.

Once they had safely removed the bead, and I woke up from surgery, the doctor came to see me.

"Why did you stick a bead up your nose Anja?"

"I wanted to see what it felt like!" I said with a smile.

I was incredibly mischievous, and very much loved by my parents and family. Lucky for them as I was going to be spending a lot more time with them as the kindergartens and preschools were finding it too difficult to manage my medical condition. I bounced around from place to place for a while, until I decided to spend more time in my parents' office playing.

I brought my plastic, fake electronic saxophone with me into the office. After irritating all the staff with the fake sax tunes, I was pushed out into the China Town Mall where there was a buzzing hub of people. I put down my hat and began to busk. I made a good $40 an hour busking that I could put into my piggy bank and got yummy Chinese lunches and the medical attention of mum and dad when I needed it. This to me seemed a lot better than kindy.

It was coming up to the time now where we had to begin looking at Primary schools. We took our 'Anja recipe' to the local Catholic private primary school up the road from our house as my parents thought I would be able to get better medical care and attention there than at a public school. I went for my "interview", and I was sweet, well dressed, brilliantly behaved and by this stage was exceeding my developmental milestones – they had no reason to refuse me, or so we thought.

They didn't want to cope with the disability so left us hanging. We knew there were places left as there were other local kids that were still getting in, but we just never got a response. By this time, it was far too late – we had given up on ever getting a response (their plan) and had to investigate other options if I wanted to be able to get in to any other school locally in time.

The public school accepted me without question. They looked after me through each "accident", excused me graciously for every doctors and hospital appointment and admission, and welcomed me into the sick bay and called mum whenever I needed it.

I was welcomed into the school by the other little kids. We had 'show and tell' and my mum helped me make a big poster on beautiful fuchsia cardboard that I picked myself, with photos of my colostomy and me as a baby in and out of hospital, and little writing about my medical condition and more pictures. I held up this poster with pride, recycling it every time it was my turn for show and tell, and told all my classmates about my little medical journey. Mum came with me the first time to help explain and make sure I was okay, but I was not phased at all and even invited my peers to see the scars on my tummy if they so wanted, which I would proudly display.

From that day on I would happily run around the playground and lift my shirt to show my classmates my scars when they asked. Even though I had occasional accidents, I would wrap my jumper around my waist and go up to the office to call mum. Everyone knew about the condition without judgement, so I didn't have to hide at all.

While I was the shining star for the days surrounding my show and tell presentations, I had myself a busy little social life. I had made wonderful friends and was really enjoying school.

On the weekends Dad was set on teaching me to ride a bike. Mum and Dad both agreed on this being a necessity, it was in my Danish blood to transport myself around on a bicycle. I began with training wheels and this was easy. Dad decided quite quickly that it was too easy, so he got out his tool kit and unscrewed the training wheels off the bike.

From too easy to too difficult, I was not able to keep upright on the bike at all. Dad broke the mop end off mum's favourite mop and thread the metal stick in through the back of my bike, so he could run around behind me holding it perpendicular to the ground (so I wouldn't face plant). I was able to have full control of the steering so learnt how to do that well, I just needed to improve my confidence and balance.

After riding around the pavement in the garden of my house, Dad decided I was ready for the road. It was a relatively quiet road, looking back definitely not *the* safest idea as cars would drive through there often enough.

Where our driveway came out there was a bit of a slope (hill) going downwards, but Dad thought it was completely fine, and assured me that he would be behind me the whole time. I trusted him, I had no reason not to (yet).

We began at the top of the hill and Dad said to start pedalling, so I did. I was flying down this hill at top speed and it felt so GOOD.

"Dad!!"

"Dad!?!?!!"

I turned to look behind me and he was standing at the top of the hill, hands on his hips looking pleased with himself, and how he was able to teach me to ride without training wheels so quickly. It was a bit premature.

As I looked behind me to find dad, I turned the handle bars and cut myself off and fell off the bike completely, scraping my leg and arm, blood running from it. Dad ran to my aid, the proud face replaced by an expression of guilt.

I was sworn off anything with wheels until I recovered so instead I spent my weekends going to zoos, medieval festivals, concerts, events in Brisbane - just having a wonderful time and an abundant life.

Mid-way through grade 1, it was time for my first sleepover. All the other kids in my grade were having them, and I was lagging behind as the umbilical cord with my mother was really short. Mum was my hero and I knew that I could rely on her to make sure I was well, and all my medical things were under control. Being away from mum for the night at this young age, despite her having travelled overseas before without me, seemed to kill my excitement for the sleepover.

Before my sleepover I had my washout and waited until I was clean. I would always have "jelly" (mucus) for the next few hours so as soon as that had stopped, and I could walk around without leaking, I was ready to go. I went to my friend's place at 5pm and we were laughing, playing and I totally forgot that I was out of the safety of my mums loving care.

By the time we went to bed, I couldn't fall asleep. My bowel was fine, so I didn't have to worry about that, but it was something else. My reflux.

It was BURNING me. I usually slept propped up on 2-3 pillows just to make it through the night, sometimes my parents had to even put my bed on an incline – with two bricks under each leg at the top of the bed, to try and help me to breathe and not be in horrible pain from the GOR.

I was too shy to ask my friends mum for three pillows, and I thought

I could make it okay on 2. When it became unbearable, I woke my friend and we got her mum to call mine, so I could be picked up.

Instead of spending nights at sleepovers, I would spend nights with my parents, going to open for inspections of houses as they were wanting to buy another investment property. Both my parents were real estate addicts and they had bred one too.

One night, after a 7:30pm inspection at a house, I gave my tick of approval as I played in the park across the road while my parents sat at the picnic table discussing the logistics.

I decided I would try a new trick and attempt to stand up on the adult swing and swing myself with my body. I thought this was a great party trick. I did it the first time while yelling out to my parents to watch over and over. I fell off harmlessly and got up and ran over to my parents, insisting they *actually* watch me this time. As they had no choice, they did.

I got up on the swing, moving my body back and forth and getting up some height. Suddenly my footing slipped, and I fell to the ground. At least my parents were watching this time. I put my hands down to break my fall, my parents rushing over when I started to cry.

My wrist *really* hurt. Mum and dad looked at it and they told me I should go to the hospital as it looked broken. I disagreed. I knew if it was broken that I would need to have surgery, and I didn't like having surgery as the gas mask would feel like it would suffocate me while I was lying flat. I would always want my mum to walk into theatre with me, but I knew that now I was old (5) I would have to go in alone.

I suggested to my parents that I was tired and wanted to go home, and they agreed so I went straight to sleep on my return home as I wanted to escape the pain. As per my usual fashion, I woke up in the car on the way to hospital around midnight. Apparently, every time I had rolled over in my sleep and bumped my arm, I screamed.

Once I arrived at the hospital, the pain was bad. They did an X-Ray and saw that I had broken two bones in my right wrist. As far as I was concerned, this was the end of my ballet career as I would miss Swan Lake!

The doctors were worried that I would keep bumping it and make it worse, so they put a cast on it to protect it until I went in for surgery.

I waited for the surgery until 1pm the following day, without any food or water as I was prepped ready to go as soon as they had time in theatre.

I was so reluctant when I got wheeled in to the operating room but was quickly put to sleep by the count of 10 with the "laughing gas".

I woke up in the middle of surgery, completely paralysed and unable to speak or move. I could see the doctors injecting me with things and pulling on my broken arm. I couldn't feel any pain, just the tugging. I was getting scared and wanted to scream but couldn't do anything. I then felt something more being injected into the IV, and I was out cold again.

V

⁘

Childhood

Don't let the situation you are in impact on your ability to feel happy

I was a very joyful and flamboyant child, and neither myself or my mother allowed my disability to hold me back in any way. I would always be so excited for different experiences, and despite needing to consider the logistics of how to manage my condition in different environments, it never dulled my enthusiasm.

When it came to my first sports day, I was very excited. I had my WO the night before and my tummy was feeling good, so I knew I shouldn't have any accidents. What I forgot, was my struggle with breathing. After my first one in grade 1 I realised that playing in the park running around was fun as I could stop as and when I needed but running in a race really sucked. I just could not suck enough air into my body and physically could not do it.

After this I was feeling run down and tired. My parents and I brushed it off as just being exhausted. It didn't get better for a while and I was starting to feel quite unwell overall. I would go to school, thinking I could make it through, and then go to the sick bay by midday to get picked up by mum.

I did this most days for a few weeks, and mum continually sent me back to school, thinking I was faking it. Even when I was sick I could still be bright, bubbly and happy so I can understand how it could seem odd I was so unwell beneath my cheeriness. Mum decided to threaten me, "If you call to come home one more time, I will take you to the doctors, that will stop you from faking it!!"

I didn't particularly like the doctors, but I knew one thing for sure, I wasn't faking it. Sure enough, after coming home early the next day I was sent to the doctors. They ran some precautionary blood tests, and mum insisted on me going back to school until we got the results.

Mum got a call from the doctor, for the past four weeks, I had glandular fever, and its expected span was another 2 weeks. I was so happy as I thought FINALLY I was able to stay home and rest.

After a few days at home, mum declared to me, "you seem much better now, back to school you go!!"

I learnt that unless I felt so sick I thought I was going to die, I wasn't *that* sick, so I should just get on with it. Adopting this mentality helped mum to realise that when I was sick, I was really sick, and for me it meant that my pain threshold and illness threshold increased exponentially, so I could function well physically even when I when I had a mild flu or virus.

Once I was over the glandular fever, things went back to being great. I was enjoying school and excelling academically.

By the time it was grade 2 sports day, I had enough of the whole "running as a competition" thing. There was no way I would go to Sports Day. I cried, stomped my feet and told mum I was simply just too sick to go. My smart Mumma had already worked out that I hated sports day and knew it was an act. Looking back, I think the fact complaining about how much I hated it for the twelve months since the previous one probably gave it away.

So, little me went to Sports Day against my will and competed in all the events. It came as no surprise to me that I did not get anything but a participation ribbon and pneumonia. That sounds dramatic, I know. From all the laboured breathing and being around other kids with colds who were breathing heavily, was enough for me to be admitted to hospital the following day with pneumonia. I really need to thank coincidence for landing me a great 'hall pass' for getting out of future sports days!

I was pleased with myself after this event, but unfortunately the issue landed me in my respiratory specialists' office once again. After reviewing scans and examining me, they proposed to my parents and I that I should get a stent put in to my air pipe to hold it open, so I wouldn't struggle with my breathing so much. It did seem like a good idea as it would resolve a big problem. After careful consideration we decided against it as we wanted to give my body the opportunity to heal and strengthen itself – the surgery was too risky.

I had approximately 50 hospital admissions under the age of 5, and more surgeries than what could be counted on both my hands. These were *admissions,* not presentations.

I worked out my own way of dealing with things – listening carefully to my body to detect whether or not I would have an accident. With my swallowing I would always make sure I carried a water bottle to wash down my food, also a great way to stay hydrated with my one kidney. If the water couldn't wash food down, I would go to the bathroom and try and throw up the food so I could swallow and breathe properly. To everyone else it seemed like I was sick, and mum got many comments about it when she would take me out to dinner. To me, it was just hospital prevention.

From five to twelve, my medical issues really settled down – with my episodes of pneumonia and bowel blockage becoming few and far between, things were a lot better with my health.

My parents and I decided that we wanted to have a more relaxed and healthier lifestyle, and we knew we could find this on the Sunshine Coast. We finally had the opportunity to move up there as I was a lot healthier by then and didn't need to be constantly close to the hospital in Brisbane.

My dad always discussed my condition openly, most times against my knowledge and will – but I am not too phased by it these days. I remember him telling our removalists when we moved from Brisbane to Coolum about my birth condition and defects. Talking to two strange men about my anus and vagina wasn't as carefree by this age as I was just starting to work out the privacy surrounding those topics. Oh well.

I quickly adapted to the coastal lifestyle, and really loved it. Mum and I spent every morning from 6:30am-7:30am before school in the ocean. I started in a new school and was already topping my class academically and made some great new friends.

Mum had been offered a job at one of the institutes on the Sunshine Coast, and Dad was going to be working from home and only going down to the office a few days each week to check in with the staff.

Unfortunately, by March that year, at the age of 7, my parents' relationship had deteriorated, and they decided it would be best for them to split up. I was very close with my mum, we always joked that the umbilical cord wasn't long enough, as I would always cry when she would have to go overseas on business trips when I was younger for 1-2 weeks at a time. I love both my parents, but my decision was clear that I would go with my mum, as her and I were joined at the hip as she was always the one by my bedside in hospital and staying up throughout the night with me when I was sick.

They got everything finalised and I went with my mum.

After the year contract was finished at the institution, mum opted not to extend as her company needed her back on board and they rented their office out in Brisbane and got new staff to work out of a home-office on the Sunshine Coast. Mum also wanted me to move to a better school where I would have better potential to flourish academically.

In classic teacher fashion, she looked up the state-wide NAPLAN exam results of all schools on the Sunshine Coast, and she found that a public school in the Hinterland was topping the results at that time. So, the decision was made – we were to move up to the Montville, leaving the house in Coolum to my dad. Despite my pleas to not move to the "countryside" where my ears would pop every time we would drive up the mountain range, it was happening.

Mum negotiated with me, so I could help to choose the house we bought if I complied with moving up there. I settled on this beautiful house in a cul-de-sac with glass looking out to a beautiful garden, one acre and lovely trees for climbing. The selling factor for me was the pink carpets, furniture and floral curtains and accessories that the older lady who owned the house had. It was a 7-year-old girl's dream. I didn't realise this would all be ripped out, so we could renovate – mum kept that part a secret.

Our neighbouring property had a view over the lake and running creek and waterfall – and was vacant land that we were welcomed to explore.

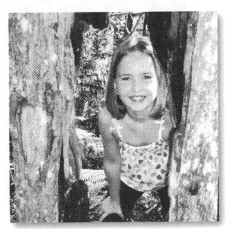

Little me on a Bush Walk

I began clearing out the old sticks, leaves and rocks from the creek and waterfall, and made it a beautiful series of bathing holes for my new friends and I (there were only 16 kids in my grade – it was great). I got a tarpaulin and threaded it through the branches of the best climbing tree on our property and made a series of hammocks where I could relax with my friends. I was finally living a great life!

I had decided not to be the "special" girl anymore and make it on my own merits.

Despite any hesitations, I started at another new school for year four and decided that I would be a bit more open to living with nature and start studying Buddhism. It sounds very spiritual saying this now, but honestly, I had just heard rumours that you could have a power nap during the meditation time and did a lot of colouring in. That said, after listening to the stories of Buddha and learning meditation I really loved it!

Speaking of rumours, one began to circulate about me. I had begun telling my close friends a bit about my birth condition. It could only be private until we started swimming in the creek together and I had unexplained scars over my body. I told one of them that I was born without a bum as I thought that was the easiest way to explain it.

I knew Chinese whispers had got out of hand when someone came to ask me if they could feel my bum, asking if it was made from the same kind of plastic as their lunch container.

I was more annoyed about this than upset about it… I just wished that people would have an awareness of what it was and understand what the condition was all about. As soon as I told a friend, within 48 hours' mum would get a phone call from their mothers asking if I was okay, or if it was all a lie. To the 'general public' my condition seemed far too serious and complex to be true and shocked the mothers to find out that both their child and I were telling the truth about it.

It added a bit of soap opera drama to my life, and I didn't quite mind it.

I had finally got to the age where school camps started. I was soooo excited for this, as I was buzzing off everyone else's excitement. By the time I had to go, I realised that I would have to manage my wash outs away from home by myself.

My mum had already taught me how to do it however often I insisted she help me. We had adapted the process to be less uncomfortable as being in a foetal position as a child can make you feel vulnerable – even when you trust what is happening. Honestly, mum and I just got over all the preparation and plastic waste with lying on the floor, so I would just sit on the toilet and lean forward and do it that way. It made it so much easier when I had to do it myself.

Administering my WOs was only part of the problem. I would be taken away from my friends for them to query where I was when I was doing my washouts.

I wasn't worried about people knowing about my condition, I just wanted to be involved in all the activities and not miss out. I was comfortable for my friends to know but having my little primary school crush know I had to be taken away to spend an hour on the toilet was a bit embarrassing to me. I wasn't worried about the condition being exposed, just that no one else had told me about their bowel movements, so why should I?

My first ever camp in Grade 4, and similarly the one in Grade 5, were very manageable. They were being held at an activities camp 15 minutes' drive from my house, and 10 minutes' drive from my school. This meant, mum could come and pick me up when we had our "Free Time" before dinner and take me home for me to do my wash outs and wait till I was 'clean', before dropping me back. This worked wonderfully for me.

I was able to sleep with the pillows that I brought with me, so I was propped up if I needed them to battle the reflux, and my bowels were able to make it through with my home washout plan.

We told the school beforehand what we thought was best for the situation I was in, and how I could manage my condition but still be able to have as much of a normal and full experience as all the other kids. They were very understanding and did what they could to accommodate me, and it worked well.

I had been making friends easily. As the school was quite small and friendly, and most classes were mixed levels. It was a close community and really everyone was your friend. I have such fond memories of asking for a rope as a birthday present, so I could weave a platform in my favourite climbing tree and running around the macadamia plantation at one of my friend's places.

Life was like I had never experienced it before – my friends and I could make little dams in the creek on the neighbouring property, so we had "private spas" and bringing picnics down to have by the fresh water. We were wild – if we needed to pee, we would just go in the bushes!! I used to be far too prim and proper to even consider this thought, but when you were a long run up the hill from the toilet, you got to do what you got to do. We were never scared of snakes, despite having seen three in the first week of moving to Montville and packing my bags and threatening to leave.

My friends and I would put up tents in our backyards and sleep there, up to eight of us girls in a big camping tent. We would build forts with sticks. I would have blisters on the inside of my thumbs from being on the ride on mower too long. I would be tanned and toned as mum decided to get 6 cubic meters of mulch dumped on our property to create garden beds with. I would have to go to the doctors to get a tick removed from the back of my skull as it had buried in too deep and I thought it would paralyse my brain.

They really were some of the best days of my life.

By the time I got to grade 6, the camp was a longer way away, and only accessible by barge. If I decided to go to it, I would not be able to be rescued by mum, unless I was carried out of there in an ambulance. I to-ed and fro-ed with the idea in my head and discussed it with some of my best friends. They of course told me I just *had* to come, because it would be so exciting, so I decided that I would trust my body, and go for it.

We were staying in cabins, about 6 of us girls to one toilet. The school insisted, much to my appreciation, that I would be able to do my wash-outs in privacy, without lots of people in my cabin rushing me or asking questions.

So, by the time we got our free time segment (1-2 hours), I would be accompanied down to the far end of camp, to a public toilet block where I was able to use the disabled toilet cubicle.

I decided to make things easier, I wouldn't have a WO on my second night.

The weather was cool and rainy, and I had got cold and wet that day, and then again, the next morning. We were walking out to the "Giant Drop" and "Pamper Pole" activities where we would be suspended from great heights on ropes in harnesses. The walk was about a kilometre from the camp or maybe more. As my bowels can react very quickly to any foods or change of my body temperature, as my body was cold and wet, I began to feel myself have an accident.

I had to get up my courage and quickly whisper to the teacher that I had to go back to the camp and use the bathroom. They didn't know about my condition like a few of the other teachers did and began questioning me until I insisted to them I had a bowel problem and just had to. I walked back to the camp, 1km in distance with dirty undies, and have them rub against me causing me to get a horrible rash. I knew that having it pressed into me for so long I was guaranteed to have a UTI by the time I got home.

Needing a distraction, I decided to start my own business. As a little 9-year-old sales person, I launched a local dog walking business and went door knocking to get clients. I had my sights set on equal success with this venture as what I had with my saxophone busking business at the age of three.

I got quite a few regular clients. It turns out wealthy, kind retirees respond well to young blonde girls willing to do their 'dirty work' for money. By dirty work I mean cleaning up dog poo on the walks I would take their dogs on. Really, I was used to cleaning up poo so I wasn't too phased. Despite my marketable $4.50/walk rate, my mother quickly felt guilty with the good, tax free income I was making and made me stop charging and do it from the goodness of my heart.

I am all about the goodness of my heart, but dad had given me an incentive to save, matching dollar for dollar, and I couldn't save without an income! Regardless, it is fair to say my dog walking business went into liquidation. What would I do next to keep myself entertained?

VI

Change

Let the bad times allow you to appreciate the good times more

Even though I had such a self-inflicted busy schedule, some weekends I would go down and see my dad. As we had not spent much time together he would always spoil me and take me fishing with elaborate picnics he would pack or take me to the circus or movies. We hadn't bonded as much as Mum and I had during my childhood as he was always taking care of the management and finances of the business.

With these great weekends together, Dad and my relationship was going really well. He had been depressed after the break-up and had just begun getting happy again and had a new take on life. His relationship with mum was getting so much better, they were speaking and could spend time together once again.

Dad decided to get laser eye surgery as he was sick of wearing retro glasses and had begun swimming in the ocean regularly. He asked mum and I to stay at his place the night after the surgery as he had to be supervised post-anaesthetic. We came back home with him and I stayed with him while mum ducked off to donate blood. Dad said to me that he had a headache and was going to go to bed and I told him to let me know if he needed anything. That was the last time I ever heard my dad speak – early January 2010 at the age of 11.

That year I was due to start Grade 7 – the last year of Primary School.

My health had been great, apart from occasional pneumonia, tonsillitis (before having them removed) and regular cystoscopies (checks with a camera under GA) to ensure that I wouldn't have any problems or retained blood when coming into puberty. I felt the healthiest I had ever been being immersed in nature. Even though I was enjoying being well, I would have given anything to be the sick one in the family if it meant that no one else had to be. I knew I was strong and could cope with it like I had many times before. Unfortunately, things don't work that way.

That one morning in January 2010 broke my heart. My dad woke up unable to speak and dropping his unresponsive right arm with his functioning left one. We gave him water and it ran out the side of his mouth. We called the ambulance and they carried him out of his house.

Mum and I followed anxiously behind the ambulance to the nearest hospital before we lost them – almost half an hour away from our house. They did not want to stress dad, so they did not have any sirens on. In my innocence I couldn't think that the issue was so serious as they didn't have sirens blazing?

The ambulance arrived at the hospital before we did. They sent dad for a brain scan. The doctors came back, and we were told 85% of his brain was dead from a huge stroke, and he would likely pass away within the few days to follow. I still remember the room it happened in – my usually strong, Mr fix-it, capable father looked so small and fragile laying in the hospital bed with his eyes closed. My mother, aunty and her husband were all huddled around his bed as a team of doctors spoke to us.

We said our prayers and shed our tears.

This was to date the most heart-wrenching experience for me.

Mum and I spent the first night in hospital with him, sleeping together in one of those fold out hospital armchairs. Nurses were in and out, running further checks, taking observations and checking on his catheter as he was unable to move much.

He managed to survive through the first few days before we began seeing improvements. The doctors told us it was a miracle however he was not guaranteed to live just yet.

Within the first few days after the stroke, my half-sister from Denmark flew over to be with us, and her, mum and I were driving 20 minutes from Dad's place to the hospital to see him. One morning I wasn't feeling very well, and my tummy didn't feel good. My mother gave me a banana to try and fix it, as mothers' first reactions seem to be "you haven't eaten/drunk enough/blood sugar is low." While we were driving, we saw this beautiful flowering tree and pulled over to pick some flowers to have on Dad's bedside. I was beginning to feel worse.

I have a high pain threshold, so I knew that having such intense pain meant something was very wrong. I told mum as soon as she got back in the car, and we agreed it was lucky we were heading to the hospital anyway.

By the time we got there I was barely able to get out of the car, I couldn't straighten up with the pain and any movement (even walking) was agonising. As it wasn't really something I could just ignore and take a few deep breaths and get on with, Mum took me to emergency.

The doctors immediately thought it was my appendix. My mum had some memory of my surgeon saying that he removed my appendix in one of the major surgeries in my early years, so it didn't cause trouble later on. The doctors treating me were unable to gain access to my medical records from the children's hospital so were unable to confirm if this was correct.

After running thorough tests, they diagnosed acute Pelvic Inflammatory Disease (PID) which is basically an infection of the uterus lining and the fallopian tubes. This diagnosis seemed almost unbelievable for a 11-year-old who was not sexually active as usually it is associated with sexually transmitted infections. At this stage I did not even have my period, so the thought of any internal contamination was near impossible.

The conclusion that was made was that due to my bowel incontinence, there could have been cross-contamination with my vagina. As my pelvic nerves are so poor, I cannot feel when I have leakage until it touches the outside surface as warmth, meaning cross contamination is plausible as I have no 'early warning system'.

As I was still so young, after getting my pain 'under control' with strong painkillers, they wheeled me up to the Children's ward rather than Gynaecology for my care.

After I had spent the night and the doctors were more confident that I was stable, I was able to get a wheelchair and go upstairs to visit dad. My family, my sister and my poor mum had to bounce between dad and I in the hospital, and the stress that would have been on mum at that stage was unbelievable. Throughout the whole thing Mum stayed strong, loving and positive.

The pain was unreal. My whole abdomen was so tender, and nothing could relieve it fully. Day after day the doctors would come past, and I would beg to be released so I could go and be with my dad and family properly. They would ask me to jump and watch my face carefully to assess my pain level. By day 4, I was able to perfect my acting, and jumped with a straight face so I could leave, despite the pain still being there.

I went straight up to the ward to my father and recommenced my position in the chair by his bedside. I couldn't fathom what karmic injustice had put my father in this situation.

He was released from hospital after 1 month and transferred to a rehabilitation Centre as he had none of his speech back and he was still incredibly weak and fragile. He had been prescribed anti-depressants, blood thinners and a further concoction of medications, including one for epilepsy. Dad had frequent seizures due to the electrical activity in his brain considering so much had died and was replaced with brain fluid.

I still had hope that he would recover… that I would be able to hear his voice again. All he could say now was "Dar dar" and "NO." When dad arrived in Rehab, the speech therapist and physios would come and ask him if he is ready to go to therapy, and he would say "no", his only word, and they would leave again thinking he really meant 'no'.

It was like my real father died when he had the stroke, and there was just a shell left. I was thankful he had made it through and was now trying to navigate the new dynamic and Dad's care needs.

By the time Dad started at the rehab centre, I was starting grade 7.

Between going down to see dad every day after school, and watching him make very little improvement, it was coming time to elect two school captains, a treasurer and secretary. How my school of 180 students (16 in my grade) worked, was all the people in grade seven who wanted to be school captain would make a speech at assembly in front of my whole school, and then everyone would get a vote.

This vote was real Australian election style – you needed to write the little number of your preferences in each box next to the candidates. Doing a speech in front of the whole school didn't even stump me – I had been making speeches at most family occasions, standing on top of whatever furniture I could find and clinking glasses, from the day I could talk.

Seven of the nine girls in my grade all wanted to be school captain and were well suited for the role. I so badly wanted it but understood how unlikely it was – I had come in grade 4, other candidates' parents were so involved in the school and broader community and had older siblings that were school captain previously.

I didn't think I stood much of a chance. My only claim to fame was in grade 5 when I performed to "Don't Stop the Music" by Rihanna, a dance choreographed by my friends and I. Us four performed together, and my top fell down mid performance exposing my breasts. Either the voters all felt sorry for me or they are a bunch of perverts, because we won the talent contest! Could this get me over the line two years later to win school captaincy?

Only one boy ran for school captain. Statistically, primary aged children will stay loyal to their gender, so I knew half the school at least would have him as their number 1 preference, but who would take the other place was a mystery.

The speeches were great, and I knew it would be a close vote.

Everyone had come for the announcement assembly, even my mum. I thought she was there to pick up the pieces of my school captaincy loss. When the names were read I was nervous, and in total shock when my name was called - "Anja, School Captain"

EEEEEEEEEEEEEEEEEEEEEEEEEEEEEEEEEEEEEEEEE – I thought this was the best day of my life. Surprise mum, you were there to see my victory! Mum had another surprise for me though... I know you are thinking a bunch of flowers, or an ice cream, but she likes to keep me on my feet, and walked me to the doctors for my Swine Flu shot. It was safe to say that I wasn't too impressed.

Soon after my long list of School Captaincy duties in the broader Montville community began, it was time for my dad to get out of Rehab. He came up to Montville to live with us and we would all go down to his Coolum house a few nights each week, so he would be in the comfort of his own home. He was still having seizures that we learnt to manage and could not communicate – read, write, speak, understand (?) at all.

It was like a high speed rollercoaster ride anticipating Dad's care needs. His medications would upset his stomach, and I would go on walks with him and he would have to stop on the side of the road and pull down his pants to go to the toilet. I was distraught and wanted to protect him as much as I could – I knew what the feeling of not being able to control your bowel was like.

We tried to get dad into other Rehab centres to improve his speech, but no one would take him after an assessment as he was unable to be rehabilitated. Mum and I tried to teach him sign language and learn it ourselves, but he did not have the brain capacity to know when to use it. We bought him an iPad and installed an app and programmed it with things he may need to say and taught him how to use it, but he still couldn't think to implement it when needed, and he thought the whole thing was a massive joke.

Being school captain was the most extraordinary experience. Everyone in the community knew me – I felt like a celebrity. We led the Opening Ceremony for a new building at the school, presented at the Great Walk festival in the community on a weekend, hosted many things and were involved in a lot of work in the community. I was delivering speeches in front of audiences of 200-300 people at the age of 11 – it seems incredible when I think I was only that young, but at the time it felt so natural.

Before I knew it, it came time for me to graduate from Primary school and discover the next chapter of my life that was waiting for me.

As the year ended, there were a lot of changes in sight. Despite the success of the business while working out of the home office in Montville, there would be much greater opportunities back in Brisbane. My mother again had assessed the options for schooling based on academia, whilst I assessed based on uniform and our top selection was a private, catholic all-girls school that had been our local one before we moved up the coast. When I was a child, sitting on the balcony on my potty, I would watch the girls from that high school run past my front veranda for their cross-country race. Surely, a sign.

There were long wait lists for admission, but I had to give it a shot. I went for my interview, and wore the most conservative, appropriate dress I could find, was very well groomed and wore my gold cross to complete the look. My mother had instructed me to look like a young, smart girl going to Sunday school before the church service, and I thought I fit the brief. I felt like an undercover Buddhist trying to infiltrate a Catholic school system.

The deputy principal interviewed me and told me that I would have to wait until September to find out if I had been accepted. If I waited that long, it would rule out my other options for high school as it was leaving things a bit late.

The week following my interview, my mum got a call from the school. They told her they had a place for me there and were looking forward to welcoming me into year 8 in 2011.

I was bombarded by book lists, and school rules, requirements – how polished your shoes need to be and how long to wear your tie.

Starting high school is bad enough, but my mum and I did not have anywhere to live yet in Brisbane. We also had to work out what to do with my father to ensure he was happy and safe, not to mention my bowel incontinence, breathing problems and frequent doctor's appointments.

We had Dad assessed for care entitlements, and found he was eligible to 5 hours a week care. This was not enough. Unfortunately, the stroke did not eliminate dad's stubbornness. In fact, is acted as an enhancer. He was too proud to have any care, so we only utilised 2 hours a week and called the care worker a "cleaner."

Dad wanted to be in his own home – his pride and joy – once again. He had been gradually spending a few nights by himself there, and we trialled a few blocks of days with him by himself, and he was able to make it through with flying colours. Dad's epilepsy subsided as his brain began to rewire, so it was much safer for him to be alone than it was previously.

We sold our beautiful house in Montville, put the money on the stock market and moved to Brisbane, staying with my family until we rented a place and got on our feet. Every weekend we would come up the coast to take care of Dad; cook meals for him to keep frozen and reheat, do extra cleaning, wash clothes, ensure he was showering okay and had everything that he needed.

When dad needed mums support, despite the break up, she was there, has always been there and will always be there. Mum was my perfect role model of unconditional love.

Mum, Dad and I threw ourselves into this new arrangement - it was all getting real, I was starting high school!!

VII

High School

Embrace all new experiences as opportunities for growth

The week before starting school, I got my period. I was not too impressed but felt like I was finally a woman. That, and I now had an appropriate excuse to wear pads for the security of any bowel accidents that could catch me by surprise. Thankfully by the time the first day of school came around, it had stopped.

Heading through the school gates, I strapped on my dorky backpack that was double the size that I was and tried to make some friends. I timidly signed up for the debating team last minute as I had always wanted to do debating, and mum said I would be great at it because "I loved arguing". What teenage girl *doesn't* love arguing?

I went to the sign-up meeting and they pulled a group of five of us timid grade-eighters together to form a team. We had amazing coaches - the previous debating captain that had just graduated and two wonderful teachers. We would have team meetings once a 6-day timetable cycle and it would be one of my favourite lunch times - we would discuss tactics and start preparing for our big debate. In the meantime, I was finding my feet in high school.

Everyone already had big groups of friends from their primary school, so it was difficult to find my tribe. I ended up befriending the girl that would sit next to me in my homeroom, and all core classes.

We became so close like sisters, speaking the same way, dressing the same, writing the same – it was amazing. Gradually we built up our own friendship group, always with the core members of myself, her and another best friend that lived around the corner from me.

Most of the girls in my group played Netball, and quickly convinced me to join in and do it too. I went and joined the netball club with my best friend who lived around the corner from me. I would wear denim shorts and a t-shirt to training as I was so clueless and had no active wear!!

It was safe to say that my netball career was short lived and disastrous. I told everyone in my team to not pass me the ball, even if I called for it as I was quite literally, scared of getting it. Unfortunately, at times they would forget the protocol and pass it to me, only for me to quickly pass it on like in a game of hot potato.

I would stand next to the WA as I was pitched as WD, and would get them leaning on me, intimidating me and pushing me away during games. I was scared as these girls were fierce, determined and quite violent. If a girl pushed me I would say "sorry" to her. It just wasn't a game for me.

After mum came to watch one of my games as support, she brought to my intention that it was incredibly clear I was hopeless at it. She was being very generous to tell me that, as I was worse than hopeless at netball.

Everything happens for a reason, and from playing netball I got my first and only trophy! It read "U14's Netball Division 3 – Participation" Mum didn't quite agree with my awesome trophy sitting on the mantelpiece, so it quickly gained a proud place on a shelf in my room.

As time progressed I got closer and closer with my two friends and began to let them understand my disability more. It was so easy to hide behind the more glamorous of the health details and hide the fact that I still had bowel accidents, and no matter what, that was not going to change. Getting my period, it became easier as I could use that as an excuse if I ever had an issue.

My close friends were incredibly understanding and supportive of me, despite not knowing the full extent of my issues as I would not let on to anyone how little bowel control I really had, as I believed then it was "too much information".

Managing the shock of surprise bowel problems was enough, but by the end of Term 1 I had another shock… my first B-. My first ever B (apart from sports as I am sure you could have guessed). I was horrified. I decided to knuckle down. I began studying crazily hard and striving that extra mile. With every assignment, my grades were improving and I slowly, assignment by assignment, exam after exam started getting back to A level.

I would be working so hard on assignments and study from the moment I got home from school. I was always making study cards, studying with my friends and even went so far as to make a study poster for a final exam for science as it wasn't one of my stronger subjects. I was determined to achieve success.

I always thought I loved science, but at my primary school all we had done was try to measure how hot it was in an alfoil box we made and didn't even get the point explained to us. So, it was fair to say that my science knowledge had fallen behind in comparison to all the city kids. I could build a woven platform in a tree with rope, but I definitely could not tell you about the forces relating to a moving object.

Every weekend without fail, I would go up to my dad's place. He was doing quite well, he had stopped having seizures by this time and had stopped his epilepsy medication. He had made friends again in the community, the newsagent thinking he was on drugs the first time seeing him post-stroke.

If you have ever met my father, you would know he dances to the beat of his own drum. We would come up one weekend, and find the laundry washed in an oat and milk-based breakfast drink as the packet looked like washing powder. We would look in his dishwasher to see what he had put in there and found the TV antenna box from his roof there. We would then go to investigate how he would have gotten up on the roof and see a "dad-sized" hole through the corrugated plastic roofing in the outdoor area, where he must have fallen through. Any suggestion of him being put into care he would be adamantly enraged about. He had horrible mood swings from the brain injury and would label mum and I as good cop/bad cop and would switch around our roles on every occasion.

Every time my friends would say anything about their father, I would get a twang in my gut because I realised the finality of never having the dad I knew, in my life ever again. Sometimes it would just hit me, and I would be overwhelmed and cry, as it is a challenging situation to be in and make sense of. I just missed who my dad used to be.

It all became real when I was watching a video of myself as a child a few years after the stroke, and there was a heavily-accented man's voice, and I said to mum, "Who's that?"… she just said, "that's your father Anja."

The more I would think about the loss of my father, the more it would harm me. It was so hard to grieve as the father I knew was gone, but the shell of him was still here. I would do anything to have been able to bring back the man I once knew. I wanted to make dad proud, so I knuckled down in my studies.

Debating with the girls was going well. We were undefeated, winning every debate of the four in the preliminary rounds and made it through to the finals!

At a similar time, I received a letter from the school saying that I had been selected for the *Days of Excellence* program for debating. This was a special program offered to the top achievers in each subject area, depending on programs being run each year. I was so excited about this opportunity and could not wait.

When the day came, I scrubbed my white hat with a toothbrush and set off with one of the other girls from my team. It was a great day with many other debaters from schools across Brisbane and the greater region. This filled me with great confidence in my ability to achieve highly in years to come.

Going into grade 9, my first challenge was the swimming carnival. Yes, you already know that I suck at swimming - most sports really – so it is an almost guaranteed disaster.

It was compulsory to do one race minimum, and I was oblivious to that fact I could have played the 'disabled' card and got out of it. I signed up for 50m freestyle because there was nothing easier and put myself in the lowest division available.

I went. I swam my race. I didn't place (big surprise). I went back up to the top of the bleachers and felt my stomach gurgle as I pulled on my shorts before my togs filled with a feeling of warmth that was all too familiar. Considering that my washouts were salty water and glycerol, a salty water and chlorine pool, cold and with added stress, 'fast' swimming and 'intense' exercise, could set my stomach off. Some days it would be fine, but that day, of all days, it wasn't.

I wrapped a towel around my waist and told my friend that I just got my period and I had to go. I had to ask to borrow my friends phone as I was still yet to get one, calling my mother for a SOS as it was at a public pool a few hundred metres away from where mum worked. For some reason, mum didn't bring the car, she decided to WALK to come and collect me.

I said goodbye quickly and ducked off downstairs, innocently thinking

I could just slip away and get out to my mum. I was stopped in my tracks at the exit by one of the teachers.

"Where do you think you're going?" she said to me in a tone of authority.

I leaned in towards her, telling her I got my period and it was on my shorts, and that my mum would come and get me, so I could go home and get cleaned up. I could have told her the truth, but I figured any woman would be empathetic with a surprise period, and much more understanding of that than a bowel accident.

Mum came and got me, and I walked along the footpath of the main, busy road, towel wrapped around my waist and my head hanging low. Bugger. Swimming Carnival 1 – Anja 0.

Much to my relief, there were more exciting things to talk about than my little disappearance the previous day... BOYS.

Most of the girls in high school had kissed a boy. Saying that now almost seems silly, but your first kiss was a BIG DEAL. Lots of other girls had kissed someone, but I hadn't.

I was so curious about it and intrigued to find the right boy to share this kiss with. Sweetly and innocently enough, I met one at a school dance, had a bit of a "high school awkward waltz" and called it a night. We began talking over Facebook and it was all incredibly exciting, but it wasn't until about six months later that we met again, went on a few dates and kissed. To be honest I can't even really remember my first kiss these days.

It was so innocent and sweet, and even sitting next to him let alone HOLDING HANDS would give me butterflies. I didn't particularly love the kissing as I thought it was too wet and slimy and couldn't particularly understand why other people enjoyed it so much. I just appreciated having someone that I could 'love' and whose company I could enjoy.

The coinciding of me beginning my periods at the start of high school, understanding what sex is and then having a boyfriend made the doctors, mum and myself realise that it was time to work some things out about my gynaecological situation.

I went to my GP (General Practitioner), the same one that I have had since I was born and got a referral to a gynaecologist. I had to see this doctor privately as she came highly recommended. My mum came with me and we sat in this small consultation room in one of the private hospitals in Brisbane talking to this lady who was unfamiliar with my birth condition.

She asked me some questions, looked through my ultrasound scans and examined me. I really did not know what to expect from this appointment.

It was revealed my two uteri were intact – both with one cervix and one ovary each. The examination was incredibly painful, with my legs up on those things like you see in movies of women giving birth. She fingered in and around the vagina, testing the capacity and feeling the rigid scar tissue. If this would be anything like what sex would feel like, I did not want any part of it.

Something you forget about surgical scars are that they are not elastic like skin, and certainly don't stretch to accommodate. For god's sakes I could not even fit a tampon in there!

She sat me down after examining me, and told me that from my reconstruction at birth, the vaginal opening had become very small and rigid. So much for mum saying, "Don't worry about it, they're like a piano accordion and just accommodate."

The gynaecologist informed me that two years before I wanted to have sex, I would have to come back and begin vaginal dilation – the same method used for anal dilatation all those years ago. Hard plastic rods, forced up inside, breaking the skin so it could grow back bigger, stretching the scar tissue with a bloody ending each time. Ouch.

I walked out annoyed and stressed, "That sounds like a horrible thing to go through again" I thought, as well as being very frustrated that I would never have a normal romantic sexual experience. Instead I would have to plan, calculate, see the doctors regularly, and have everyone, including my mother, knowing and controlling when I could lose my virginity!

There would be no spontaneous flame of passion and romance, a four-poster bed with white, see-through curtains overlooking the ocean. To be honest, I wasn't even sure whether or not I could *have* sex. I put it on the back burner as it wasn't something that could happen at that time.

Navigating my sexuality was coming into play. More people (doctors) had seen my genitals than those that have seen the bits of the local prostitute. The fantasy and sexuality of it was stolen from me very young as it became something I associated with the "medical" world – one I desperately wanted to get away from! I would have doctors touch and examine me from the day I was born to the current day... they have touched everything, been everywhere, nothing has been left unseen. Anything sexual couldn't even be on the cards after these constant experiences.

Sex didn't cross my mind until other people in my grade started having it, and there was pressure put on me by my then boyfriend. It was pushing me to my limit as I knew I had such a limited capacity, and after everything

I had been through with my reconstruction, I didn't want to lose it in a time or way that I would regret.

I really knew I was so different. I was quick to adapt to a "no sex before marriage" mentality. It was easier that way. I was not able to have sex and thought it would be more acceptable to show it as a strong respective belief rather than an inability.

I knew that I was an emotionally driven person, and my sexuality would have to develop from my emotions rather than hormones.

Anyway, there were more pressing things on my mind for now…

VIII

⚬⚭⚬

Persistence

*Take every emotion and experience as a directive to show
you what way to go*

I was finding year 9 a lot better than year 8. I was working hard academically and getting good grades, was in a great new class with some wonderful new people and my friendship group expanded.

I joined the school choir, placed 28th out of approximately 160 at cross country and was selected as class captain.

My studies were going so well that at the school's awards night I was presented an "Academic Achievement" award and I could not have been happier.

Things were really beginning to go my way, and I went into grade 10 confidently, choosing Science, Maths B, French and Business, as well as my other core subjects. I was in classes again with some great people and was elected class captain for a second time.

While I was breaking my back academically, my mother decided that I was still a bit too "country" and needed to go to etiquette classes. There was nothing wrong with my etiquette at all in my mind, just that sometimes I would not cross my legs when I sat down and would speak in slang.

So, in July 2013 I went to study a "Diploma of Professional Modelling" with a strong focus on etiquette. It wasn't a "real" diploma but covered everything I needed to know. We were taught how to walk in super high heels, talk, dress, shake hands, do our makeup and hair, pose for photos – everything. I was so thankful to Mum for preparing me so well for the future.

After doing well on the catwalk at the graduation, I was talking to one of the people in the modelling school who invited me in for a meeting.

Before I knew it, Mum and I were in their offices where I had done my modelling training and I was having my meeting. We talked about everything, and they said that while I was still in school and with such a heavy academic load (all OP subjects – Maths B, Chemistry, French, Bio and more) it would be hard for me to go to the necessary castings or get too much work as I would only be available on nights and weekends.

They also asked to check if I had any scars. I confessed that I did and was requested to show them. The kind lady told me, as compassionately as she could, that I would never be able to show my stomach in any photos or castings, and that would cut down the work I was able to do significantly.

Apart from those things, she said if I was still interested after understanding that's the way it would be, she was happy to set up another test shoot for me and go from there.

Another test shoot? Never showing my stomach? My dream was Victoria's Secret, the same as hundreds of thousands of girls out there. The thought of never being able to achieve that dream and hiding my scars as they weren't considered "beautiful" was confusing to believe. I did not feel like my scars could or would hold me back from modelling, so it was a strange "reality check".

I walked out of that office numb. I really did want to do modelling but didn't realise that having scars on my stomach would be so unacceptable. I thought people were becoming more accepting, understanding chronic health problems and if not all of that, there is photoshop! If I said I wasn't disheartened, I'd be lying.

I sent a few of my photos to several other modelling agencies and after seeing some poorly lit and angled bikini photos of me, scars and all, I got a few rejections. I hated to admit to anyone that I had been rejected as I had always thought I could achieve whatever I set my mind to. It became a bit of a sensitive topic for me, and I tried to stay as far away from it as possible as I did not want to be rejected again and was still shakily building my confidence.

With that going along in the background, I knew that I would always have a career open to me based on my academic merit. I began doing more to follow my heart and became actively involved in the St Vincent De Paul

Charity Group and would go to the aged care home as often as I possibly could, based on the roster.

I had another huge reward for my achievements when I was selected for *Days of Excellence* once again. This time, it was for both Biology and for Debating – and I spent two days at each of these. They were both incredible days and I felt blessed and privileged to be one of two girls from my year chosen for these two areas.

I had met a lovely guy out of a coincidence, through friends. We had become very close and began dating. Just a few months ago I had decided to be on my own for a while and focus on myself, but the most amazing people come into your life when you just stop looking for them.

He was always in my corner from the beginning. I told him about my issues and he respected and agreed with my decision to save sex until marriage. He understood the journey I would travel to be able to have sex and to not rush that process. We were both still young. As soon as school holidays began he was flying over to Europe for a month with his family, so we began making plans for early January when he would return home.

Before I knew it, it was the awards ceremony for grade 10 and once again I was invited. They lined us all up, we practiced standing together and walking together once again.

That night I did my hair beautifully and was ready to go, still unaware of the award I was going to be receiving.

"Anja– DUX – Business and Academic Excellence Award" - Wow. I never really thought that I would pursue business (despite really enjoying it) and I could not believe that I had come first in that subject. I loved achieving academic acclaim and was joyous to know that I was the highest achiever in that subject area. I quickly found out that Academic Excellence was a step up from Academic Achievement and was so thrilled that I had been progressing positively.

As I was doing so well, I knew that I would have all study options available to me. For a long time, I had my sights set on pursuing a career in law and politics or medicine. I knew medicine so well because of my experiences, and I thought I was already half qualified. I have a great sense of human justice, empathy, upliftment and serving others and at this time I wanted to do something 'well-respected' that would make a difference to people's lives and pay well. Due to the instability of the health of my body I always would seek financial security.

My mother's side of her family are very academically oriented having all had incredible careers. Being 'smart', working/studying something prestigious and earning lots of money are seen as signs of superiority to them. This is really the case in society when you look at it carefully. I have been in that mindset too, so I can't judge it. But with an amazing thing called perspective that you get from being a sick child, I think superiority should not even be a thing. And if it is, shouldn't it be judged on love, kindness, human decency and strength when overcoming life's obstacles?

Unsure of what to do just yet, I was constantly a high-achiever, I put so much pressure on myself and the wheels were beginning to show signs of falling off.

I was quite wound up. I had such high expectations of myself and had the complete confidence to achieve whatever I set my mind to. I was always pushing myself harder and higher, nothing was ever good enough to me unless it was the best. When I would get back a B+ rather than an A and when I wasn't seeing enough improvement from the gym I would beat myself up about it as I knew I could do better.

This was causing a lot of tension at home as I could not tolerate anything I perceived as judgement, so when mum would offer constructive criticism it turned into a battlefield.

Mum, with love in her heart, knowing that we both just wanted some time away from each other, booked me flights to Denmark, to go over there for a month in my school holidays.

This would have been an amazing gesture to anyone else, but in that situation, I felt powerless as I had not been consulted on the decision and had made plans with friends and my boyfriend for over the school holidays. Mum had booked tickets for me to go to Denmark on Boxing day, all by myself, and return home the day before starting grade 11.

When I got told, despite knowing I would love Denmark and time with my sister and her little family I was not happy as it meant my boyfriend and I did not see each other for two months, and I was flying overseas by myself.

I enjoyed the few weeks of school holidays in Australia with my friends before my trip. One day I went into the city to meet one of my good friends to shop and eat lunch.

We walked through the city, hopeful we could find a potential dress for our semi-formal that was about three months away.

Before I knew it, I had been scouted by the manager of one of the stores, whose wife designed the wedding dresses. I tried on dress after dress, modelling each of them worth more than my life savings tripled. I had a taste of the modelling I had been yearning for however was still concerned that my scars would hold me back as that is what I had been told.

My best friend and I went and got a celebratory Boost juice, cheers-ing it in the air as we sat in one of the food courts in the city. I couldn't have asked for a better day - I got a taste of what I really wanted to do in life, be a model (and a bride– but that's for another time).

As soon as I got home I emailed the man, and he returned an instant response, thanking me for the day and telling me that he would be in touch when they were planning to shoot the campaign. The shoot was likely to be the following year in April - four and a half months away.

In a flash, I was on the flight over to Denmark. As the flight was beginning its descent, the air hostesses moved me to first class as I was an unaccompanied minor and they could let me out of the plane first easier. Arriving in Copenhagen in style, I couldn't wait to see my sister, her husband and two children.

I was having a beautiful time in Denmark. My sister and I would go out on runs together in the mornings when it was crisp and cold – snow lining the streets - and I would lag about 500m behind her at all times. After that we were quickly launched into party preparation mode as my sister was hosting a New Year's party - a tradition she had of throwing the best NYE parties for years.

The boys stocked up on fireworks and my sister and I decorated the tables, as per her careful design instructions.

As it got closer to midnight, the boys were outside testing some of the fireworks. There were little popping fireworks that you could play with on the ground, and I was amazed my sister's young children were so comfortable and familiar with how to handle themselves with fireworks and could even set them off by themselves – a very common occurrence in Denmark.

As we counted down the new year, it dropped past zero degrees and I was eagerly anticipating seeing snow for the first time. We all got up on chairs, tables and sofas. "5...4...3...2...1... HAPPY NEW YEAR!" We screamed, jumping high off where we were, and landing on the ground with a thud! A Danish tradition for "jumping into the new year" or maybe it was just my sister's tradition, I never quite found out.

We went out into the cold, crisp midnight air and set off some fireworks from the centre of the lawn - my sister and I holding onto each other's arms, so happy to be together for the new year.

She took me upstairs to the balcony and we looked over the roofs of Danish houses on a flat horizon, the whole sky filled with amazing bright fireworks clouded with smoke, coming out of everyone's backyards simultaneously. It sounded like bombs being dropped but was one of the most breathtaking, magical sights I have ever seen.

My sister and I came downstairs eventually and were saying goodbye to most of the guests as they were filing out. We decided together that our New Year's Resolution would be doing a 1-minute plank every day to try and get abs - something we both wanted.

At 2am on New Year's Day, we were on the floor doing our first plank.

As the days passed by, I was having a brilliant time. My sister took me out to get the best burgers at her huge local shopping centre. We had just ordered and were sitting there in this funky burger joint and just enjoying each other's company with great anticipation for the food. Just as we received our food, we looked out the window and it began to snow! My first time seeing snow despite being back to Denmark multiple times. Every time I had been in Denmark previously was during the summer months to avoid me getting a chest infection from the cold weather. We quickly scoffed down our food and ran out into the carpark, so I could experience it.

My sister filmed, as I walked around in amazement – catching snowflakes on my tongue and being amazed that each little piece of snow had its own delicate pattern. I couldn't believe the beauty that was in front of my eyes.

I had seen a funny photo on Facebook paying out a girl who took a photo in the snow in her bikini. I thought it would be a great, memorable photo, and had brought bikinis specifically for this purpose. We raced home in the car and I ran inside to put on my bikinis and snow boots. I ran outside with my sister in tow, taking a million photos and laughing at this "crazy Aussie girl." One of the neighbours had a daughter almost my age that I got along well with, and we took the funniest photo with her all rugged up for the snow and me standing next to her in a bikini -both of us laughing.

The snow was beginning to get thicker and line the streets like a cake sprinkled with icing sugar. I went and put on my snow clothes and went out into the snow - going for a walk down the street. The neighbour and I tried to make a snowman, and took photos lying next to it. It was beginning to get cold and I was glad to be rugged up under many layers.

We went back to her house and she showed me this flying fox that they had made that carries you through the air across their backyard. I was anxious at first but after encouragement, I climbed up to a platform and got on the flying fox.

I flew through a backyard of snow, the winter air nipping at my cheeks.

I was having such a brilliant time in Denmark. As I was there for a month, my sister had arranged for me to be a guest teacher in my eldest nephew's English class as well as many other adventures with her and other family.

Not wanting to leave, I was back on a flight home to start Grade 11, my most important year of schooling yet. I felt hopeful and confident for the future. I could see nothing standing between me and my happily ever after. Yet.

IX

<hr>

Unravelling

*Depression and anxiety occurs to tell you that you are going
in the wrong direction or focusing on the wrong thing*

From the moment I walked through the front gates of school, my feeling of anticipation succumbed to one of distress. I had already put an overwhelming sense of pressure on myself. I loved learning and succeeding, however really wanted to be able to do it all without such extreme stress.

In every spare moment of thought, I would be antagonising myself internally about something. Whether it was having too much fat on my thighs, breasts that were too small, a friend that I had a tiff with or an assignment I was worried wasn't perfect.

I was playing a continuous tape of self-criticism with no stop button. Everything that I did not think was perfect, wasn't sure how to approach or didn't *really* want to do, would play on my mind constantly. I was in my super sensitive teen years.

I would go over in my head how I was going to do each thing – what I would say in a situation, plan out every second of my day to ensure I got one to two hours of gym into my afternoon as well as my homework done, assignments and even extra revision for each subject not to mention my WOs. I would exercise until my shoes filled with blood from blisters and didn't feel like it was making a difference to my body. If I had to make a phone call to someone I didn't know, I would have to write down what I was going to say before calling up.

I had perfectionism laced with anxiety. I had been putting so much pressure on myself, that every teenager – or really even every person on this planet – is guilty of doing.

The semi-formal was quickly approaching and I was thankful my sweet boyfriend could come with me, so I didn't have the pressure of needing to find a date. I did however have the pressure of wanting to be in amazing shape and looking fantastic. I had eaten a lot in Denmark but stayed in great shape running, and with my sister's and my New year's resolution planks.

I was increasing my workouts - doing an hour-long weights class followed by an hour of yoga and Pilates, I would also do step classes, running, cycling and weights. If I hadn't gone to the gym, I would not be happy with myself.

I went to a dietician to get a good diet together. They tried explaining to me I wouldn't see the results I wanted from the gym if I wasn't eating and fuelling my body as I was in a pattern of starving myself thin. I wasn't even thin, which was the most irritating part – no matter what I did, or what weight I lost, I would still look "healthy". It really was a blessing, but I could not see it that way at all.

My body was run down physically and mentally, as I was working out in the afternoon/evening and I was staying up until after 1am studying.

Semi-formal was the huge talk at school, and despite being just as concerned as everyone else, I had my mind in the clouds. Choosing the jewellery and clutch, booking in makeup, hair and tans, just even more added pressure.

By the time it came around, I found the experience to be far more stressful than it was rewarding.

One night in term 2 of year 11, I was just so overwhelmed I broke into tears. Everything was too much. My dad, always having to manage my disability, friendship politics and the stresses I was putting onto myself with school. I cried to my mother and was scared realising a state of anxiety and depression had really snuck up on me. That was probably one of the most normal problems I thought I had - it was normal right? Everyone at high school then seemed to be impacted by varying levels of depression and anxiety.

My upset was completely self-inflicted, and I just was not feeling great. I knew by the morning I'd be feeling a lot better, and it was just a 'boo-hoo' moment. I knew I had to get myself together as I was a strong person, physically and emotionally, who was just stuck in negative thought patterns that caused a heightened anxiety.

After that night, mum insisted I stay home the next day to get on top of my school work and have a moment to myself. It was a "mental health day" mum insisted.

I woke up in the morning in my pyjamas, tied my hair back and put some oil on my face and swollen eyes. I sat in the middle bedroom of the house where the computer was, working diligently on all my assignments and doing extra homework and study, while mum was at work.

A peaceful day ended with police cars at the front of the property as a man had come trying to kick down the front door while I was home alone. This was my complete worst nightmare since I was a child. He had broken the locks on the downstairs door and was seconds away from getting in just before he got sprung. He was trying to break in.

If I wasn't stressed and overwhelmed before, I sure was now.

That night, mum was shocked as I told her the story. She could not believe that I had responded in the way I did (crawled into a corner facing the wall and shaking) and didn't defend myself or barricade myself in a room. Of course, we did not have any locks on the bedroom and bathroom doors, so it wasn't as simple as closing and locking a door. I didn't want to do that because I knew then the man would know I was inside, and scared.

Mum taught me how to barricade myself in her room. Moving the chests of drawers, other heavy things and securing myself. This should have given me some sort of relief, but it just instilled the fear in me that it could happen again, and the man who "let me get away", with the icy blue eyes, would come back with a vengeance.

The next day I turned up at school and was pulled out of class unexpectedly. The school counsellor wanted to speak to me after mum had sent a concerned email to the school without me knowing, expressing concerns after my distress at what had happened.

I would go to the school counsellor once a week for three to four weeks, talking about it over and over, relaying every detail until it was stamped with a hot iron into my brain. The more I talked about it, the more I focused on it. She was a kind, compassionate lady, and gave me techniques to cope, relaxation tapes and did all she could to help. Five minutes by myself, home alone, while mum was picking up milk would leave me hiding, shaking and purely terrified.

It took around a year, before I could be home alone without freaking out, and about 14 months after the incident we ended up moving to a new house. That day had really scared me and added to my stress in a way you couldn't believe. I no longer felt safe, and my home was no longer my sanctuary.

I realised the counsellor was unable to help me, and the change had to come from me and the belief I could protect myself, and not focusing on it happening it again.

By the time the June July holidays in year 11 came around, I was eager for a break.

My aunty had a tradition of doing something special with my cousins and I during our holidays, as it wasn't often we all got to spend time together. I was almost 16, and my other cousins were 14, 12 and 11. We were all girls, and loved spending girly time together.

My mum confiscated my phone, and I went away with my cousins, aunty and uncle, to a horse ranch about 4 hours north of Brisbane. It was a cute place, and we had two days of horse riding planned. Spending time with my family was really what I needed after all that I had been through.

It was a wonderful getaway – the horse riding, despite a bit scary and my horse being stubborn and deciding to stop, run or to jump over logs whenever he felt like, was beautiful. We would go out on long trails and stop by little creeks and have a snack. The only downside were these HUGE mosquitoes that were easily bigger than the size of my thumbnail. We were getting bitten everywhere, and by the second day drowned ourselves in insect repellent to try and keep them away.

By the time that I went back to school for Term 3, I was feeling on top of things.

Mid-week of the third week back, I began feeling unwell. My stomach felt really unsettled and knowing that this could lead to some accident I went to the sickbay and was collected by my mum. She completely understood and took me home.

In addition to my tummy feeling unsettled, I felt generally weak and tired. It was only week three back, so I couldn't imagine it would be stress induced, or exhaustion.

The next day I went back to school, and I was okay, and made it through the rest of the week. The following week I made it to Tuesday before needing to be picked up again. I was feeling weak, dizzy, nauseous, tummy gurgling, abdominal pain and very ill. *Something* was not right.

These rare occurrences of me being picked up from school during the day were becoming more frequent, and I was beginning to need to take more and more days off in a row. I was falling behind on school work because I was missing lessons and tried to catch up as much as I could online, but it is not the same as being in class, and much harder to do when I needed to be in bed. As I still wasn't comfortable at home, I had to set up a bed under one of the desks in my mum's office. Sit up in the chair and try to do some school work, and then be so hit with exhaustion that I would have to lay down.

Days turned into multiple days, and multiple days quickly turned into weeks. I would feel a little bit better as I had been resting and go to school and push through the day. I had to go and speak with the Principal of Academics about my situation. She was very compassionate but didn't fail to highlight to me that as it was year 11, missing some of the units would impact on my university entrance level.

As soon as I realised this illness wasn't my birth condition playing up, and wasn't going to go away without action, I hopped onto the medical merry-go-round.

I started with my GP, who ran a multitude of blood tests, that all came back without any flags apart from Adenovirus and an Iron Deficiency which couldn't account for all the symptoms that I was experiencing. Symptoms were flaring and pointing at a full body condition. She could take my temperature, and I had a thermometer at home too, and every day without fail I would have a low-grade fever. There was no one that could pull this all together, so I was referred off to different specialists that would be able to investigate what was going wrong.

Firstly, I had developed tachycardia (racing heart), which is common to accompany bradycardia (slow heart). The differentiation between my slow resting heart rate, and when I suddenly had racing was enough to send me spinning and sucking in breath. My GP thought this was reason enough to send me to a cardiologist and wrote a referral and I was seen quite quickly.

After running tests, they were unable to find anything conclusive that could explain what I was experiencing.

I was also sent to the gastroenterology clinic as my stomach was gurgling, I had a mix of diarrhoea, constipation and bleeding, and unexplained abdominal pain.

They thought the first step would be a scope under general anaesthetic, and next a full colonoscopy a month or so later, also under anaesthetic. They took biopsies and they all came back clear. They could see some irritation and little tears from where the enema was pushed into me daily, but apart from that, nothing that could explain my symptoms.

I went into the clinic at the hospital to get my full results and a treatment plan and waited for just over two hours before seeing the doctors for a 10-minute discussion – if that. The doctor, unfamiliar with Imperforate Anus or my condition, was unable to help. It was made clear that he had not read through any medical history of mine from the moment he opened his mouth.

The doctor told me that I had issues with chronic constipation - something that I knew. He suggested to me that I take daily laxatives to keep my bowels loose and moving through. My mother and I both reiterated to him, that due to my condition, if I had laxatives I would not be able to function, leave the house and let alone go to school, as I had no control and had to have social continence. He couldn't quite understand this. I told him a story, of me having a few strong laxatives and nothing happening, until unexpectedly THREE days later I had a bowel explosion. There was no way I could even *try* this regime and be able to live a functioning life. Besides, I knew this was not the cause of my illness.

Mum and I walked out of that office, and realised we had just wasted months of time, and exposed me to anaesthetics twice for nothing.

I was referred to gynaecology too. They are wonderful, and I love my gynaecology team that I still see to this day. They are incredibly compassionate and accommodating. They did a CT scan and found I had a 5cm haemorrhagic ovarian cyst on my left ovary. Thankfully, it was able to resolve itself however I was often getting reoccurring cysts on that ovary.

One of the gynaecology team's key concerns was that I was now in a relationship and had not begun vaginal dilation. I told them my technique of saving my virginity until marriage, but they were persistent for me to start now as they could see that it would be a long journey ahead.

When I went back to the clinic they did a thorough examination, finding that my vaginal opening was still the size of my pinkie and unable to fit a tampon in, and that it was an incredibly rigid opening. They wanted to test my capacity and find out my anatomy exactly. No matter how many ultrasounds and CT scans I had, they found it very difficult to identify where everything was.

They stuck a very long swab, 'ear bud' type utensil inside my vaginal, taking it out and measuring it. It had a bit of blood on it as it was so tight and tender. They found my right cervix was only 5cm in from my vaginal entry, and the other 11cm up after having to veer left.

They introduced me to these hard-plastic rods that would soon become a part of my daily routine. The smaller one was a comparable size to a mini-tampon, and when I would have to push this in it was so painful and would sometimes bleed. It would bleed when it would break the skin and stretch it, and as it would irritate the sensitive cervix that was tucked in so close to the opening.

I was given some lube and steroid cream to use when I did my dilatations, that I had to aim to do at least three times a week. This was during the period of time I was still unwell with low-grade fevers.

Mum and I also discussed with the doctors my urethral-vaginal fistula, as when I would pee it would come out in two streams. I still would get constant UTIs, so we thought perhaps this fistula could be contributing to it.

I was referred to urology to get this explored, and I knew even as a complex case, it would take a few months for it to be processed. These were months of illness I couldn't afford to experience.

As no one could work out what was going on with my body, my GP referred me to a Physician to get some fresh eyes on my case. Apparently, a Physician is like a specialist GP that could help to pull everything together.

Mum and I ventured to his office and unfortunately, despite him being an amazing doctor, he was unable to help.

I was missing more and more school, and it was adding to my stress levels. I was just getting sicker and sicker. I was beginning to lose all my muscle tone and strength. I went from a girl who would go to the gym two hours a day, four to five times a week, to not even being able to sit up as my body could not hold me and I would be in such horrible muscle pain and general fatigue.

I thought I had exhausted all options. I knew that my schooling had been affected detrimentally by this mystery illness, and what annoyed me the most is that I was feeling terrible and I couldn't give my sickness a name. I felt without this label I couldn't justify to myself or others why I had missed so much school or be able to give a time period for recovery.

A month or so earlier in July, I had gone to an Education Exhibition with my best friend. This was where all the universities, colleges and academies would come together and set up stalls, and you could walk through and talk to their team of staff, ask any questions and get brochures for their different programs.

I had bags full of brochures from the top university in Brisbane for Law and Medicine. I had collected information packs about the medical entrance exam and was sitting in the car of the way up to dads, with my mum driving as I went through all the practice questions. I had no idea that in a few months to come, I would be questioning if I could even finish high school.

We arrived at dads and had my mums best friend from year 8 coming over for dinner with her partner. She had moved from Western Australia and my mum hadn't seen her since they were in school in 1968. They had recently got in contact and I was excited to meet one of the people mum had such fond memories of through school.

As soon as we met, we got along well. I always enjoyed being around adults as growing up in hospital and spending a lot of time in my parent's office and work functions.

My mum's friend, Alex, was telling me that she could see I was becoming unwell from signs in my iris, face and fingernails, as she had been trained in naturopathy, iridology and Chinese face reading. I wasn't aware of this side of medicine, as I had always been in and out of hospitals, had my symptoms treated rather than the cause, and been pumped with antibiotics, painkillers and a whole array of medications.

She gave me some suggestions of what I could do, and that at that stage it was important to get a balance of good gut bacteria, have lots of yogurt and start on some enzymes. I was so grateful for her heartfelt care and advice and could feel in my body that I was becoming unwell. She quickly resumed the position of 'aunty' or 'god mother' as she felt like my guardian angel from our first ever meeting.

What held me back from doing what she told me, was an obsession with a diagnosis. Such a strong drive that would stop me from treating the illness myself naturally as I wanted to be able to justify how I felt to others by giving them a medical name they could look up. I thought also with this diagnosis the doctors would know how to treat me adequately, and that all those medical professionals that said they couldn't see anything wrong, and even some people close to me that didn't quite believe how sick I was because I was so good at faking being well, would be proved wrong. This was an ego trip, that cost me my health for a long time.

I concluded eventually, that it wasn't so much the doctors wouldn't help me, but more they couldn't. I could run to doctors to my heart's content, but it would not make me better. I realised that it was never and is never a doctor's responsibility to care for our health and prevent us from suffering illnesses. The responsibility falls with us.

Once I knew that the responsibility was mine, I knew exactly where to go. To my godmother.

X

Choices

You never need a reason to do something more than "it feels best" – trust your intuition

I was desperate. I had about 1 week to decide my future, and it was all depending on when I was "cured" back to health again. The school was putting pressure on me to decide what I was going to do. It was getting close to the end of the term and it was clear most of my assignments were unable to be done because of how much I had missed. Similarly, being able to sit my final exams was less likely than seeing the tooth fairy.

I understood I wasn't going to experience a miracle, but at this stage I was needing some relief. I was so weak, so dizzy and so exhausted. My weakness had turned into a fully body pain, every muscle and every joint would ache without end. My abdomen was sore and painful. I was still bleeding from my bottom.

I went to my godmother and spent most of the weekend with her and my mum. She told me about topical use of Castor Oil, and how there is so much research supporting it dissolving cysts and scar tissue. She told me the story of her friend who was told she would never be able to have children due to her polycystic ovarian syndrome (PCOS), and she began doing castor oil packs each night and ended up falling pregnant. She proceeded to have an easy pregnancy and a beautiful daughter as all the cysts were dissolved by the castor oil.

It was obvious from my scans that I had reoccurring cysts on my left ovary, and a given from all the surgeries I have had that there would be masses of scar tissue. I didn't realise that scar tissue could be a cause of abdominal pain, something I was experiencing constantly. Bowels, periods and scar tissue are a cocktail of things that don't mix well.

I began doing my Castor Oil (topical use) packs straight away and had immense relief from the abdominal pain that I was experiencing daily. Mum got into it too as she was limping around from a Bakers Cyst behind one of her knees, and Carpool Tunnel syndrome in her wrist that was looking like it would need surgery. In a matter of weeks, her cyst had dissolved completely, and her wrist was feeling great with no need for surgery at all.

I also started taking large doses of enzymes. This really helped with my muscle and joint pain and took it away within a few days. It also is good at eating scar tissue, so helped with my abdominal pain as well.

These two things alone improved my condition dramatically. I was still experiencing low grade fevers, weakness and exhaustion, but a huge portion of the pain factor was now removed.

This weekend was a pivotal moment for me in many ways. It would change the way I saw my health, the responsibility I decided to take over my body – emotionally and physically, and my education path.

I had been trapped in my own head thinking about what I was going to do. I didn't really enjoy high school all that much as the amount of stress and pressure, and girl politics was just a bit silly. I loved my friends, and I didn't want to be held back a year to catch up or do staggered subjects, so I would graduate the year after I was originally supposed to and have all my friends leave without me.

I wanted to study law or medicine, and knew I needed high results to be able to enter either of these. I knew that if I continued back in my grade, my OP (overall-position for university entry) would be sacrificed, and my predicted high score would take a huge hit. I had missed some of the units needed and would have to make it up by going on biology camp with the year below me while I was in year 12 and complete extra assessments when the unit was available.

The academic load already was high enough without having to complete extra units. Knowing my OP would be decreased because of what I had missed in that term, and having to make it up another time would make things very difficult. I also didn't know when my weakness and fever would go away.

I found it hard at first to shake the anger that I had been studying at school for ten and a half years, and after missing 1 term my schooling career would suffer so dramatically.

I was unsure of what to do as I had so many conflicting feelings; doing what was best for my mental and physical health, following the academic footsteps of my family, working out what would create the most successful future for myself. I knew what felt best, but I was conflicted with the thought of being a "high school dropout" or a "failure".

Mum and I talked about my options, and as she is an education agent she knew of some foundation courses that I could study in a university environment that would gain me university entry. With this option I could have more time to focus on my health as it only needed four hours per subject contact a week, and an expected six hours of study per subject in our own time.

Still there were downs to this as I would never graduate high school. I thought people would treat me differently thinking I haven't finished school, I would never have a senior formal, wouldn't see my dear friends as much, another new start and environment with no familiarity, and having one of the signs of normalcy for people my age, not there anymore. It would be a huge leap of courage and show that I am taking a bet on myself and taking things into my own hands as a mature young adult.

I remember exactly where I was when the final decision was made. I was sitting in the backseat of my mums red Peugeot, looking at the backs of mum and Alex's heads and trying to get up the courage to ask for some advice, as Alex had adopted the role of being my life coach and mentor. I knew she would be able to give me a fresh perspective on what she thought would be best for me from her heart, as she has always had such a clear understanding and perspective of me as a person.

I squeaked out, "Alex," and she turned around to look at me, "Should I drop out of school?"

"*Yes*" was her only reply.

I knew my mother would always support my decision but hearing it from someone else really reinforced that I should do it. It was a bold move, but I had no hesitation in that moment or any moment since that time, that it was the decision that was perfect for me.

I filled out the forms needed and told my high school. I had to meet with the careers counsellor at my school, and she fully supported me and agreed that it was 100% the right decision in my situation.

I needed to have completed grade 11 to gain entry. The school wrote a letter for me expressing I was an outstanding student and my situation, and I attached my high-achieving report cards from the previous year. I was contacted close to straight away to say that it wouldn't be a problem and I had successfully gained entry to the Certificate IV Tertiary Preparation Program.

It cost less than my current school fees and it offered me the flexibility that I needed.

I had to decide on the course that I would want my Foundation to lead on to, so I would choose the right pre-requisite subjects and I could automatically have a place in that if I met my academic requirements.

I knew a career as a doctor would be great as I would be able to care for my patients with the empathy that I wish the doctors were able to express to me. I had a lot of experience in hospitals, surgery, diagnosis and treatment from what I had been through personally, that I thought it would be a good place for me to fit in.

As medicine is a postgraduate degree, I had to study a bachelor's degree first. I thought the one that would set me up best would be Bachelor of Nursing as I have known in my hospital experience that the nurses know a lot of the same practical and theoretical aspects that the doctors know. My maternal aunty who babysat me as a child was a nurse, and I had been exposed to many over my years in hospital. Knowing how valuable these women (and men) were in my life inspired me to want to give back in the same way.

It was settled. I was going to angle my studies towards nursing, choosing a spread of maths, biology and chemistry, similarly to what I had studied in high school. Looking for another elective to throw in the mix, I chose marketing as I thought it would be a useful skill in all areas of life.

I began preparing for another new beginning.

To my shock and horror, mum informed me that it was against university policy for people to wear high heels to classes. I was NOT impressed. I was dragged out to the shops by mum to get some flat, sensible and comfortable shoes – my least favourite kind (at that age!).

With some dorky new shoes, it was time for me to go to orientation.

I began my course in mid-October 2014. Despite relief of some of my most bothering symptoms, I was still quite unwell. I was so exhausted, and so weak. I seemed to have lost the strength in my muscles from being bed-bound for a few months. I almost lost the motivation to get out of bed altogether really. I had no energy so the thought of exercise was far from mind.

At orientation I was quite nervous. I found someone to sit next to and stuck on to him like a stage 5 clinger. We had many talks and got lots of the clerical matters sorted and learnt how to enrol in our subjects. I was amazed that this was my new environment, in a university, the youngest there and immersed with students from different cultural backgrounds. I was relieved to finally be responsible for my own academic achievement without any pressure from external sources. Trust me, there was enough pressure *inside* my head.

In my first (summer) trimester, I only selected two subjects to study so I could still focus on my health and recovery. I chose Chemistry and the core English as I thought it would give a good balance between challenging and easy.

By the evening of the first of two days of orientation, I knew that there was something wrong. I had developed severe abdominal pain. The pain centred around the lower left side of my abdomen near my hip bone, where I knew my left ovary and left uterus were squashed up.

This had developed gradually over the past week since my previous gynaecology appointment. My normal gynaecologist wasn't there, and I was referred to another gynaecologist for this visit. I went in for a check on my progress with vaginal dilatation.

I was taken behind the curtain and lay down on the bed, spreading my legs wide and bracing for the discomfort to follow.

"What dilator are you up to?" the lady asked.

"The second," I squeaked, "but even the first is still uncomfortable."

Each dilator goes up in size in terms of width and length, so it was painful to dilate the thinner internal passage as well as around the scar-tissue-webbed entrance. It was daunting to look at the first dilator size, and look at the last one. I knew I had to achieve that difference, but seeing them in comparison was like seeing the city of Brisbane, and then the country of Australia. That is not achieved in one day.

The doctor put a dab of steroid cream on the tip of the second dilator. Usually when I did it at home, I would coat the length of it with thick cream, so even the sight of such minimal usage made me wince.

Before I could ask for more, the dilator was pushed inside me. OUCH. I told the doctor that it was hurting already, and she reminded me that it was supposed to. Of course it was *supposed* to hurt. But this just hurt at the upper end of my pain tolerance. After so many procedures as a child, my pain threshold is incredibly high. So when I say it hurts a bit, it really means it is unbearable.

"STOP" I yelled to her as the tears began to trickle down my cheeks. She just held it there. I was told to breathe through the pain just keeping it there was breaking my limits. I had to get this *thing* out of my body. The doctor encouraged me to push through the pain and just leave the dilator there to stretch my insides.

"Please, just take it out" I begged her.

She did as I asked and pulled the dilator out, with blood smeared all over it.

Was it my fault? Should I have been more clear about the level of pain I was in? Was I overplaying the pain in my head? Was I supposed to just shut up and take it? It was for my own good after all...

I felt horrible. It wasn't even an experience I could talk about to anyone except my mother. I never wanted to do dilatation ever again. I knew I had to have sex some day and it was the only way to get there, but I was feeling slightly more than *discouraged* by this point.

Straight away I could feel pain in my lower abdomen. I continued to find blood in my underwear until the following morning. Once the bleeding had stopped I felt relieved. That was until another 24 hours had passed and I began to leak a yellow puss. I ignored it, and got on with things until that next week, the second day of orientation, when I was barely able to walk because of the pain in my pelvis.

I let the organiser of orientation know I could not come on the Tuesday as I was unwell. They knew my situation so weren't concerned by it. That evening we drove Alex's partner up the coast to their home from Brisbane airport. I remember sitting at the airport and clutching my sensitive abdomen. Every step I took was very painful, almost identical to what I had experienced when my dad had his stroke.

That night we stayed at dads. When I woke in the morning, I could not cope with the pain any longer. Honestly, I couldn't even walk without being in agony. Old habits die hard, off to the hospital I went.

You guessed it, Pelvic Inflammatory Disease *again* - this time from an internal 'damage' that became infected. I was in hospital for the next three to four days, landing me only a weekend away from beginning my classes. I couldn't possibly continue being so unwell that my new study path was compromised as well!

Once they had made the diagnosis they put me on IV antibiotics and wheeled me up to the ward. Being 16 now I was too old to stay in the safety of the children's ward, so I was moved to the maternity ward. My mother and the Wardy were SO amused. They parked my bed out the front of the wards for photos, with my big heat pack and bedding cushioning my stomach, giving the perfect illusion of a pregnant belly, with the huge "MATERNITY WARD" sign above my head. Mum encouraged me to put the photo up on Instagram and I captioned the photo "The rumours are true" producing great reactions to amuse me for yet another boring hospital stay pumped full of morphine.

Unlike the children's ward, the maternity ward did not have free TV. I discovered there was only one channel available. This was the maternity channel that teaches you how to bathe your newborn, and what temperature to keep them, how to hold them, when to breastfeed them. I became a mum-expert as the mothers stressed and babies cried in the beds surrounded me.

When it came time to leave the hospital, we had to go back to Brisbane and I made sure that I was ready for uni.

This could be considered my fifth school change now, and you know how I feel about those.

I was at an age where I knew how to manage my condition very well myself as I learnt to read my body's signs and respond accordingly.

I made a friend in my chemistry class, a lovely girl from the Middle East and we really hit it off. I was quite open with her about my condition, and she had Irritable Bowel Syndrome so could really understand it. Everything was going well, and I was enjoying my classes, made a few friends and was really loving my time there.

One day I had to go up the reception area to hand some forms in. I was getting sick of my flat shoes every single time I would come in to uni, so I decided to ask the receptionist why they had this rule. She just looked at me and asked me where I heard that from. I told her my mother.... and she said that there was no such rule and I was able to wear absolutely whatever I liked. I had been totally tricked!!

Now it was perfect. This decision was the best one I could have made for myself at this time. Unbeknown to me there was yet another huge decision for me to make, and it was waiting right around the corner.

It was a beautiful November day and my life was great. I did think it was great... despite still having fevers and feeling weak, I was happy. I had learnt that there was no reason for me to be miserable, and focusing on the illness would only attract more of it into my life.

I would pass this graffiti on one of the concrete walls in the valley on the way back from uni each day. The spray paint read, "whatever you focus on expands." This was one of my favourite sayings and acted as a reminder each day that focusing on the negative things I felt - emotionally and physically - would only make these issues a bigger feature in my life.

I understood that everything happens for a reason and is a crucial part of a bigger picture that won't always make sense to me when I'm standing right in front of it. I chose to perceive everything that happened in my life to be an indicator of what direction to follow. Life doesn't happen *to* you, it happens *through* you - your perceptions, beliefs and thoughts create what you experience.

I was discussing all of this with Alex, while sipping tea underneath a beautiful mango tree in her luscious garden.

"So, have you decided what you're going to do after this course, Anja?"

"Well, I'm not sure yet," I said, "I'm stuck between two options"

"What two are they?"

"I am trying to work out what the best undergraduate degree to lead into medicine is. I am stuck between nursing and paramedicine, but more leaning towards becoming a paramedic"

She laughed. She knew me far too well for the bullshit I would make up to tell myself, to ring true to her.

She blurted out in a fit of laughter, "Are you delusional darling? You are scared when a bird flies near you, how do you think you will deal with someone spurting blood out of their neck?!"

We discussed the options I had just presented... I was someone struggling with illness and a very low immune system, for life, that wanted to work in a hospital? Did I understand that people come to the hospital when they are sick, and could easily get me sick as well? Did I realise that my nervous system doesn't respond well to another person's suffering, so if I worked in an ambulance going to accident scenes I would be emotionally shaken by it? Did it make me happy to think I would be cleaning up blood, vomit, urine and poo from sick people, and watch them suffer and even die?

After understanding all of this, it was very clear that doing nursing, paramedics or even medicine, wasn't right for me as a person, my body or something that would bring me great happiness and joy.

Suddenly I felt like the image I had of myself in the future disintegrated, and at first, I was filled with nerves at what I was going to do. What really made me happy?

Alex sat there, as I suggested option after option. Most of them could be dismissed in 30 seconds as we went over what was involved in each job. As we analysed each of them and what the role entailed, if I did not have a smile on my face or a glisten of excitement in my eyes, we knew it wasn't the right career for me.

Suddenly I just burst out, "I JUST WANT TO BE A MODEL, BUT I CAN'T BECAUSE OF MY SCARS!"

XI

⟿

Passion

Take the most logical step towards your dreams rather than feeling disappointed that you cannot achieve the end goal immediately

One and a half years later it had boiled up. I hadn't realised how badly modelling was what I wanted to do, and how blocked I felt by being told I would never be able to show the scars on my stomach.

At least we found my passion, right? Fashion and modelling. Just what could I do about it? Would I ever get there if I didn't believe I could – something so deeply ingrained in me at this point.

Alex asked me if I would consider a career in fashion rather than modelling - if I could take modelling out of the picture and focus on the fashion side of things. It still made me happy. I was disheartened about the "no modelling" idea but invigorated once again with the thought of working in fashion altogether.

I am not a designer, drawer or artist. I could sew – at a B level according to my grade eight home economics for one semester. I loved clothes, was resourceful and could dress myself well – but I had no idea where to begin.

Alex and I began talking and dreaming. She told me of these parties she used to go to, the same business model as a Tupperware party. You would have a party with friends, have some nice nibbles and drinks and have the product you wish to sell being showcased. In my case, this could be racks of unique clothing that I had designed, altered or embellished. I had always wished that I could design my own clothes and have a wardrobe filled with beautiful individualised pieces.

The idea was sealed, I was going to take the leap and do my own thing.

I started off buying fabric and sewing – I first designed, measured and made a 'picnic' dress out of red gingham. It was halter neck, with a full skirt and tied at the waist, made with cotton which is good for the energy levels in your body. I didn't have the skills to do zips and elastics as I had never learnt, so I just started doing a few simple things here and there - using ties to escape the need for anything more advanced.

I had my cousin's 18th birthday coming up and I wanted to wear something beautiful to it. It wasn't until February, but I wanted to start early and perfect it. Brainstorming what I could create, I began to experiment. I then found a love for beading. I loved Bollywood movies as a child and their gorgeous saris, skirts and dresses. I thought things that were hand beaded were the epitome of elegance and beauty. "Why can't I do this?" I thought.

Well I had never tried, so why not give it a go!

I knew my family may not support this dream of mine, so I wanted to be able to quietly and gracefully show them I had talent by wearing a piece I had worked on. I knew then if they liked it they'd say it, and I could tell them I did it.

I purchased a little white cropped top, beautiful mixed coloured small beads, a needle and invisible thread and got to work. I didn't get taught to bead by anyone but managed to work it out for myself. I diligently applied myself to threading each tiny coloured bead and securing them, one by one.

Doing this inspired me to bead other pieces that I could get in stores and online. It would mean everything would be totally unique, and I had found myself to be quite good at it.

I even beaded a feature section on a simple cotton dress for my mum to wear to a family wedding.

I decided that I should now look at doing this party clothing business Alex and I had talked about.

Alex was incredibly supportive, and we worked together. She would help look online for clothing packages and we would buy them and go through everything. I would add a few beads here and there and do some alterations.

We found a beautiful Airbnb house near Brisbane City, with a pool and lovely downstairs area and began communicating with the owner to see if he would allow me to hold a small fashion event there. We booked in a day, and I invited just under 10 of my closest friends from high school.

I still had a great love for modelling, so I decided that if people don't want to try things on, they can get a sample of what it would look like if I was able to take photos in each. So, what I did was get my poor boyfriend over to my house and we shot our own little 'lookbook'.

He ironed a white sheet while I did my make up, and then we hung that up over one of our cupboards and put some heavy things on the top of the cupboard to hold the sheet up and moved every lamp in the house to be in front of our little makeshift studio to provide lighting.

We took photo after photo, of all the pieces I had to sell. I was sick and almost fainting between each shot, but apart from that was really enjoying being in front of the camera and playing the model role.

The photos turned out well, and I got them all printed and pinned them on to each coat hanger with miniature wooden pegs.

I made a beautiful non-alcoholic punch and put drinks and little snacks out for everyone.

Everything was perfect. I had made sure it was perfect. I had the help of my boyfriend, Alex, mum and my two closest friends.

I almost cancelled last minute as I was so unwell. I could barely stand up, I was weak, dizzy and feverish. It was at the stage where I was bordering on needing admission to hospital. I couldn't let my health come in the way of things now. I drew on my inner determination, I put on a smile and got strength from doing what I loved.

All my closest friends came and there were seven of us, having beautiful drinks on the deck by the pool in this modern inner-city home. There was a great playlist, and everyone was dressed up beautifully. I was so grateful for my friends support with this brave new venture of mine.

Girls were trying on clothes in one of the downstairs bedrooms, taking photos of each other – it was just a beautiful atmosphere and I sold about half of the stock I had there.

I felt so in the zone, so happy and proud of myself for taking the chance and doing it. It was a bold move, one I probably would have been fearful to make without the support of my mum, boyfriend and Alex. If I hadn't been encouraged to find and follow my passion, it all never would have happened.

I had a sense of success and accomplishment from the fashion party that I held. I did not break even, but it didn't even matter, because I loved what I was doing, and it was implanting in the world my desire to have a career in fashion.

Riding on the high of this, I felt invincible. I knew that if I felt happy emotionally, surely my body would have to follow suit and begin feeling better physically. Our cells are affected by every emotion we experience, so you can imagine that if your feelings are negative, your body would be affected physically. Disease (Dis-Ease) is only the lack of ease, comfort and happiness with where we are.

I knew by cleaning up my negative and anxious thoughts, and following what brought me joy I would become the healthiest version of myself. A positive mind frame was the best medicine for my body.

I had to be patient with myself. My body was still recovering from years of negative thought patterns, stress and teenage insecurity.

Having a chronic illness, let alone a birth malformation, I needed to ensure my physical being was set up to receive the healing I was sending it, and that there were issues from previous surgeries that would stand in my way.

I was referred to one of the top urologists in the hospital, and was very glad to be under his care. It was quickly decided that I needed to have a voiding cystourethrography (VCUG) to assess if I had a fistula between my vagina and urethra, and where it sat. I would pee in two streams so knew something wasn't quite right. The medical imaging is done by inserting a catheter through my urethra into my bladder and injecting dye. They would then remove the catheter and ask me to pee (into a cup/bucket) while they take x-rays to see the path the urine takes.

To me this sounded quite uncomfortable, but if it could save me having a constant UTI I was willing to do it.

I went into the radiology clinic at the hospital in the morning and was taken into the scanning room, dressed in a gown and removed my undies. They understood that I had complicated anatomy and rubbed a local anaesthetic cream on my genitalia.

I had catheters in many times as a child but had never had one inserted while I was awake. I braced myself for the uncomfortable feeling of unknown people fiddling with my bits and pieces. "Private Square" - they used to teach us in Primary school, was not something of existence to me.

The first nurse tried to insert the catheter. It was pressing in all different areas, and I could feel something irritating inside me. It seemed to not fit in, and for the nurse to just be probing the outside of the skin. I really did not know what was going on as I had a 'dignity sheet' over my knees so I couldn't see what was happening.

The nurse was looking a bit concerned and informed me that she was having some difficulty getting it in, and for me to just relax as there was no reason for alarm. She ushered in the radiologist, who had a look and an attempt, but no success. They were so stumped that they began putting it in near the vaginal entrance, as there was a small dimple appearing like a hole there. It quickly slid into the vagina. There was a new nurse on board, and four people huddled around me, trying to probe wherever they could.

Discomfort morphed into pain. As my nerves aren't great I couldn't tell where the catheter was sitting or being put into. Suddenly I had a near-excruciating pain, and it felt like a little pop in my body. I didn't make a noise, but I winced my face slightly, mirrored by the guilty looks on the medicos faces. It really felt like they had just penetrated my lower cervix and were trying hard to pull it out again.

The tube came out of me in another painful pop, and they told me they weren't confident enough to put it in, so called down two of the best nurses from the urology clinic, who had been putting catheters in to complex patients for the last 20 years.

The nurses were very quick and came down straight away. You could see the frustration on their faces as it was clear they thought the team that were unable to do it were incompetent. They moved everyone aside and checked that I was okay, and then started fiddling around with the catheter once again. By this stage, every little movement they made hurt.

After another 40 minutes fiddling around, trying to push it in wherever they could in any and every possible direction, they told me they were unable to do it, and they would pass the message on to my specialist for him to decide what's next.

I wiped myself off with the help of a male nurse and could see that I was bleeding. He told me that as they had fiddled around so much, they had to give me a strong antibiotic injection in my butt to ensure I didn't get a horrible infection. He stabbed the needle in and injected its contents, leaving my bum sore for the next few days, and a little purple bruise and dimple to mark the spot.

I came out of that appointment and mum was frantic, as she knew it was a very simple procedure and it had been close to two and a half hours. She had been asking reception to see if everything was okay, but they didn't tell her anything, so she was left to wait anxiously. I gave her a hug and told her my experience in the car on the way home. She was completely shocked and confused, relaying to me what my surgeon had told her about my urethral placement in my reconstructive surgery. I told her we just had to wait and see what happens.

Before hearing back from the urology team, I went to see my gynaecologist. They read through the report, and I was right – they had in fact penetrated my cervix accidentally with the catheter. The gynaecology team were so confused as to how it was so difficult to find my urethra. They got me in the examination chair with a spotlight on me to have a good look.

They were very amused. They could see what appeared to be my urethra *easily*. They let me know that the urology team had contacted them, and they were planning to do a catheter insertion under general anaesthetic.

In addition to coping with my medical appointments and uni, I was still determined to focus on a career in fashion. I was developing my skills – finding, buying, beading and altering a formal dress (top and skirt) for one of my best friends and beading a dress and making a black lace pull-over for another friend.

Quickly, I went in for my catheter insertion under GA, had the scan and went into clinic for the results. They told me that the scan was still quite unclear, and they were unable to really tell about the fistula, but they had another hypothesis about the two streams of pee I would see.

It turns out, when I was under general anaesthetic, they had a lot of trouble with insertion of the catheter too. Even my gynaecologist struggled with it, and they both had to do some investigation. What they had found was that *somehow* my labia minora had fused, and my urethra had grown to be inside my vagina. They were unable to offer any explanation of this, but they could offer a solution.

They could see that some of my vaginal entrance was being blocked off by this web of skin, and that where it had joined had formed a 'tunnel' which meant that when I peed, it would hit this barrier and go out either sides of this web of skin. This also explained why the little 'tunnel entrances' looked like my urethral openings.

Finally, we had an explanation for my constant UTIs that would just never go away, there was bacteria being trapped there that caused contamination back into the urethral passage. They arranged for a surgery to divide the labia minora to prevent this bacterial petri dish.

The surgery was booked for the 30th of March, only a month away. I was a bit hesitant as it was now years since I last had anything cut and stitched up again. I knew I had been through so much worse, but that didn't stop me from being apprehensive.

In the same spirit I held as a child, I knew that this surgery would help me, so I would always put on a smile and go into it, with the trust in my doctors that they would do the right thing.

A week after the catheter insertion under GA, I woke up in a pool of liquid, watery faeces and blood. I was shocked and horrified. I could not feel a thing and was not even woken up by it, as it was a liquid I didn't feel anything in my stomach or even the warmth while I was asleep so deeply. I had experienced this kind of thing as a child, but it had been years since this happened last. I was sixteen now, and bed accidents aren't things that any of your friends have at this age!

I yelled for my mother and she recognised the acidic smell immediately. It was overflow. Something that only came out when you were really, really blocked up in your bowels and a motion that can easily be confused as thinking that your bowels are clearing.

I cleaned myself up, and stripped and soaked the bed sheets, and then got in the car with mum to go to the hospital.

They weren't very kind at the hospital as they didn't really understand the IA condition as they had never met anyone with it before, let alone really heard of it as more than a brief example in the textbook - if even that. They thought I was just another person who was too lazy to go to the toilet and got blocked up. Not a nice way to be treated, but I had stopped relying on people really understanding my condition a long time ago.

They did my millionth abdominal x-ray, exposing my poor little ovaries and organs to further radiation, to confirm what we already worked out– that I was very blocked up.

I couldn't even feel that I was constipated, I had no idea. There was nothing different about my bowel habits, diet or food consumption, my stomach wasn't protruding in any way, but yep – sure enough I was blocked up completely.

They sent me home from emergency with a combination of laxatives for me to take. As I knew there was no way I was going to be leaving the house in the next few days, Mum and I went up to my dad's and bunkered down.

XII

Taking the leap

Have your eyes open to the opportunities you create in front of you

I was frustrated at the thought of being bathroom-bound for the next few days. Consuming such heavy laxatives would leave me nauseous, vomiting and weak. Wanting to create 'lemonade' from the situation, Alex suggested I view it as a metaphor of "getting the shit out of my life".

They say your clearest intuitive feelings and best ideas happen on the toilet or in the shower as you pass less judgement on your wild ideas, as usually you are more 'relaxed'. I decided to adapt this mentality as I ran back and forth to the toilet, my biggest focus on getting there in time, and letting everything run out of me. Sitting there, I was so free of all thought and concern about my future as I was in the moment trying to keep my body upright as I swayed with cramps and nausea. Without my guard up, I was about the receive the sign I had been waiting for since I was 14, right there on the toilet.

I was scrolling through Facebook, something I hadn't really done for months. As I was swiping through, I saw a suggested page to like. It was from this local modelling agency in Brisbane that was only two years old at the time. I had not liked any modelling agency pages on Facebook, so how did they know? Were they just collecting my google data, or was it a sign? I decided on the latter.

The post that was featured in this little box that appeared on my feed advertised an open model casting on March 29th. You had to send through your age, height, size and two recent photos of yourself. All the photos I had of myself were with longer hair, as only a week before I cut my hair to shoulder length – new hair, new me. I needed to send a photo through asap if I wanted to attend. I knew a photo taken now, with dark bags under my eyes, white-pale lips, bloated stomach and blotchy skin from the laxatives would not be appropriate. I sent the only one I had, of myself in front of the city view from the French Film Festival a few days before.

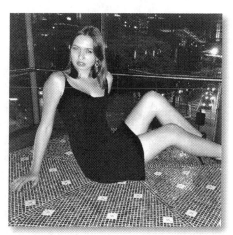

The photo I sent through

I thought I looked great in this photo, but now looking back at it from a modelling perspective, I am full of criticism. I sent the photo along with my details – all while I was sitting on the toilet. I quickly got a response back, saying that they were looking forward to meeting me. It was probably the standard response they sent to everyone, but I was thrilled and encouraged by it.

I was so happy – I had a modelling casting and my bowels were being cleared out. This casting had mysteriously popped into my news feed, and despite it being advertised for months in advance, I saw it exactly 1 week before it was happening. This was alignment.

I began my visualisation while I was laying down between running to the toilet. Visualisation had become a daily practice of mine, something Alex had taught me.

I used to be a person that would stress over the issues of the day before going to sleep, and it would keep me up at night tossing and turning. Now, I would visualise what I wanted every night as I fell asleep and found myself sleeping soundly and waking up happy. I was encouraged even further, when my visualisations would spring into reality – the power of focus, enjoying in my imaginations and positive thought.

I took the casting to be another example of the huge desire I had expressed of wanting to be a model.

I visualised walking into the casting and trying to push my energy and presence into the room. My confidence had been building quickly, however I would still find myself anxious in some social situations. The difference between when the anxiety would stop me from doing it, and that moment, was a belief in myself and a feeling of worthiness. I believed I deserved to be there.

I knew that even in moments where I had self-doubt, I should adapt the persona of the woman I wanted to be – a supermodel, a role model and someone who was sure in herself. The more I adapted to the personality, the more I adopted it fully until it became natural.

I was assured in my visualisations and played the tapes in my head of talking to the agency, doing my runway walk. I began creating a 'portfolio', grateful that I had all those photos from the fashion party 'lookbook' I could use. I would never have known when I was taking them, that I would be sliding them in to a big black folder to take with me to a casting.

Waking up the next morning, I felt fabulous. I had taken all the prescribed laxatives and felt cleaned out. My stomach had returned to normal. I was planning on going to visit Alex with mum that morning, so hopped into the shower with a huge smile on my face. I was genuinely excited for the future.

I came out of the bathroom and was chatting away to mum who was drying up some dishes in the kitchen. I was waiting, ready to go. Suddenly I had a sharp pain shoot through my chest. I thought it would just pass and was trying to relax, but it was just getting worse. I told mum and she encouraged me to take deep breaths, seeing if it would pass.

The pain intensified. I was on the floor, grabbing at my chest, gasping for breath. Mum always forgets that when you call an ambulance they can commence treatment and care for you on the way to hospital, so she thought if we left to go now we would get there a lot sooner.

As soon as I arrived at the hospital, they were rushing me into a bed, doing ECG's and giving me pain killer intravenously. My ECGs were fine, I didn't think that it was my heart as it was mainly centred around the right side of my rib cage, despite flickering over to feel like a crushing feeling across my whole chest at times.

Tears of pain and distress were streaming down my cheeks. My body was in excruciating pain, one of the worst that I had felt in a long time. I had no idea what was happening as I had never experienced anything like this before.

The doctors had no idea what to do, or what was going on. I don't recall too much, apart from getting IV fluids and the ECG monitors stuck to my body. They did no scans until much later. I was grey, could barely keep my eyes open and was really struggling. In that moment (without seeming like a drama queen) I really thought that I was going to die.

They kept squeezing injections of morphine into my drip that would spin me out. I would feel like I was floating on a cloud. It would only dull the pain for 30 seconds to 2 minutes before it would return just as strong.

I was scared. My mum was scared. The doctors were scared. No one knew what to do. They could not work it out.

My medical team contacted the other hospital to get my medical records, and once again were unable to get much. They were able to see I was in hospital in Brisbane a few days earlier and assumed that I was still blocked up with the same constipation. They were so confused at what to do with me that they diagnosed my issue as constipation. None of my symptoms linked to constipation and we reminded them I had just been fully cleaned out by magnitudes of laxatives over the past few days. The doctors could not see past my IA and treat me like a normal patient and do some more diagnostics. Constipation it was.

The plan they made, was to stabilise the pain and then put me in a medical ward for observation, while they cleaned my bowel out... again. Because they decided it was constipation, as I was writhing in pain they were trying to refuse me strong painkillers as it would concrete my bowels.

I was in a horrible, excruciating state for 10 hours before it subsided.

After this shift in pain level, they sent me up to the ward and started me on Coloxyl and movicol again. I was not allowed to eat *anything* as they were so determined for me to be fully cleaned out without putting more on top of it – even though we had told them that I had just had a bowel cleanout myself at home.

I was in a ward with a shared toilet which is not great for someone with no bowel control. I would get so little warning that I had humiliating accidents in the hospital bed and had to try and run to the bathroom after organising my drip, having it drip down my legs and needing a shower.

After two days of this, all that was coming out was clear water. I was not a happy girl, totally over this hospital stay and ready to check myself out – now only five days before my casting.

Sunday came around in a flash. It was finally the day. I got up, put on my tight jeans and white singlet, and went along to the casting. I had decided that I wouldn't talk about my disability, condition or my scars. I didn't want attention to be drawn to it, not to get in because of the scars, or only get in because I had scars and was "special." I wanted to get where I wanted to be on my own merits, without any exceptions made for me.

As I walked into the room there was a long table down the end, with David, the modelling director, Mary the booking manager and the agency's resident make-up artist. I walked confidently down to the table, introduced myself with a smile and joyfully shook everybody's hands. I spoke about my little modelling experience, why I wanted to do it, what areas I was particularly interested in and what goals I had.

I told them about my ability to travel, my freed-up schedule and my enthusiasm to take every opportunity that was given to me. I didn't mention being in hospital once a week for the past three weeks, or that I was due to go in for my surgery to divide my labia minora the following day. I was just happy in the moment.

They asked me to change into my bikini and come in to get some photos taken. I did as I was asked and watched carefully for any reactions to the scars. I acted like they didn't even exist, didn't try to hide them and aimed to shine with confidence.

The next morning, I was still buzzing. I got a call in the morning from the hospital to let me know they had an emergency case and had to postpone my surgery and would contact me again with a suitable time.

The agency told everyone we would hear from them within 24 hours. I was counting this down on my clock, with such anticipation and butterflies in my stomach. They had finished the casting by 5pm so I was waiting for that time on the Monday.

No email.

I refreshed again, still no email.

I began feeling disheartened and called Alex up to tell her about it. She told me, "As you haven't got the email yet, right in this moment, do you believe that you have got the contract? Do you *feel* that you have been chosen?"

Well the answer after being stood up by an email is a *"no not really feeling like I have got it"* and I knew that believing this and feeling this would ruin it for me. If I had a chance of getting it, it wouldn't happen if I lost belief in myself now. You must *feel* something first before you will create it in your reality. You can never have anything or experience anything that you cannot imagine.

If I could not imagine getting into the agency and couldn't believe I could, it was almost a guaranteed 'not going to happen'. By checking my emails all the time and seeing that I hadn't got one, I was focused on lack.

Alex gave me the realisation that I needed, and I put my phone down and went to bed. I visualised the email. I visualised getting the contract and signing it. I visualised the feeling of being the supermodel and walking down the runway. I visualised how excited I would be and the celebration I would have knowing I was now part of a modelling agency. I felt the great feeling and I believed in myself.

I went to bed that night at 10:15pm. I got the email, with the contract attached, at 10:30pm.

I received the development contract that I needed – a 3 month one that was given to most of the beginners to see their commitment to modelling. I knew I had commitment, drive and passion, and all that I was waiting for was for someone to take a chance on me.

I had a huge sense of accomplishment and pride that I set my mind to something and I did it. It didn't matter that I didn't have a shoot yet, I was just so happy that I was given a chance.

Within a fortnight, the agency hosted a runway and posing training for all the newbies. I was so excited for this and went along as my usual happy self.

Our training was taught by this wonderful Model who had her big break walking New York fashion week. She was such an inspiration to me and I could not stop looking at how beautiful she was, and how well she could walk and pose. The team from my agency was there as well as a talented fashion photographer, John.

I worked so hard on my walk and posing that day and made big improvements over those few hours. We each had to do a walk individually – the best one we could do, and everyone needed to vote anonymously afterwards for who had the best walk, and who had the most improved walk. I was blown away for my peers to vote that I had the best walk! I just could not even believe it was all happening.

A few days after this, I had my first ever photoshoot with one of the other models I was signed with. It was unpaid, but a great experience for us, and was being organised by one of the top stylists in Brisbane – an opportunity that we couldn't miss. We were told to wear glamorous makeup and curl our hair.

There would be a hair and makeup artist there for touch ups, but to save time we had to come with it done. We needed to wear something bright and fluorescent, or pastel colours from our own wardrobes as it was a campaign shoot for one of the nice hotels in Brisbane, at night.

I grabbed a fluorescent orange jumpsuit from the clothes that I had left over from the fashion party and a few extra pieces I had bought in anticipation of holding another one. It worked out perfectly as it was the only thing that fit the brief that I had in my wardrobe.

I went into mum's office in the morning and did some study. Mum was going to drop me there at 4pm as I still had my learners license. I realised when I arrived at the office for the day, that my black high heels had some scuff marks on them. I knew well enough that it was unacceptable for a model for have scuff marks on their shoes. I started to panic, not knowing where to get shoes in the little time I had left before needing to be there.

I quickly thought of the op shop around the corner, and dashed up there, finding the perfect black shoes that fitted me exactly, for only $10.

I did my makeup beautifully, the Diploma of Modelling that I had done really paid off well. Now it was time for the curls.

I cannot do hair. My mum, who has never done her hair or worn makeup in her entire life, could certainly not do hair. I didn't have much choice than to let mum give it a go and try to instruct her how to use this thin curling wand I hadn't used (successfully) before.

When this hot wand was in mum's hand, it was like giving a child a new toy – her eyes just lit up. She began curling my hair, that was just longer than shoulder length that this time. "Anja, why is your hair smoking?" she innocently asked me.

Apart from burning my hair she was quite good at it, with all the curls forming into ringlets, falling in front of my eyes, I thought she was on the right track. She curled my little bangs back off my face, and all was great.

I went to have a look in the bathroom and oh my god. I looked like little bo-peep with hundreds of ringlets bouncing ABOVE my shoulders. Crap.

I quickly got my brush and tried to brush it out into Victoria's Secret waves. This didn't quite work out for me and I needed a miracle. I looked like someone pulled out of a disco in the 80s. It was not quite the seductive look I was going for. I tried watering it down and it only improved the situation *very* slightly.

Despite that setback, I arrived on time. I looked like I had been swept up in a tropical cyclone on the way there. The hair stylist made some improvements, enquiring as to who and how my hair got into its current state, leaving me awkwardly blushing.

The shoot itself was amazing – on a beautiful pool deck in the evening. It couldn't have been more picturesque.

I had such a wonderful time and felt like I was in the exact right place for me, for one of the first times in my life – I was just meant to be there. That is how it feels when you find your passion, and I had not only found it, but I was living it.

I learnt to always be prepared – perfectly groomed and ready to shoot at the drop of a hat.

After the hotel campaign I felt in the groove and was selected for three shoots in that next week - two portfolio ones set up by my agency, and one TFP (time in return for photos – unpaid) highly styled shoot with a great photographer on the Gold Coast. I loved every single one of them and was blown away that it was little old me in these photos!

I felt like my life was suddenly all lollipops and rainbows and could not believe that I was me, every day that I woke up. I felt clicked into purpose.

XIII

❦

Living my dream

When you feel joy, you attract the opportunities you have
desired in order to experience more of that emotion

There really was no better feeling than confidence. Made up beautifully with professional hair and makeup, I looked like all those other models I would see on magazines, social media or on TV. I was assured I finally belonged, and I was able to achieve whatever I set my mind to. I believed in myself without ego or arrogance, which I felt was the key for me to get wherever I wanted to go in life.

My confidence was growing exponentially and the furthest thing from my mind was my chronic illness and birth condition. Modelling seems super easy, and as much as it flowed I was surprised at the amount of hard work involved. You had to prepare for weeks before each shoot - exercise, diet, personal grooming, the financial investment and the training and practice in posing and runway.

It was all coming together quicker than I could have possibly imagined.

The following Monday I woke up to a message from Mary, my manager, who amazes me as she seems to work 24/7 and had been arranging a shoot for me in the early hours of the morning (2am). She asked if I was available to shoot with John, a photographer that was also at the first runway training I had done. Of course I said yes, excited to work with John as I had adored some of his previous images with other models and was overjoyed that he had expressed interest in doing a shoot with me!

I pulled together some clothes from my wardrobe in the genre that I could never quite understand the style of, "Street Style". I grabbed some scarves, shorts, tops and jumpsuits and was ready to see what John and I could come up with together.

We took a series of great photos – John and I were getting on so well, he was shooting from the right angles and we were both suggesting great ideas. We had a few outfit changes where I could incorporate my styling skills, and my skills really developed throughout the shoot. John warmed my heart, describing me as a "natural".

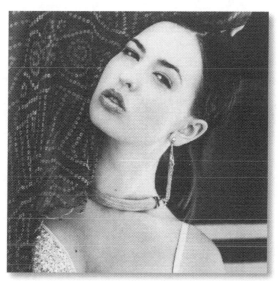

My new headshot - photo by John Pryke

A few days after this shoot marked 1 month into my 3-month contract with the agency. I hadn't got back many photos (if any) from the other shoots I had done as they were still being processed, but John sent me a folder with a large selection of images from our shoot that night. He also sent them to my agency.

I was nervous to open the images as I am usually overly critical of them, and very particular with what ones I like best. To my surprise, I could not fault them! I loved John's work and working with him in general so was very pleased there was such a good result.

Shortly after, I received a message from David, the director of my modelling agency saying that he was incredibly pleased with my dedication, commitment and results. He had received praise from everyone I had worked with, especially John, his close friend. David and Mary proceeded to tell me that they wanted to extend me to a 12-month contract as soon as my three-month development one finished. I was overjoyed. I could not have asked for better news.

John, an incredibly experienced photographer who had worked in media for over 30 years, photographed princess Diana and was very well respected in the Brisbane Fashion Community commented on the new profile picture of my modelling Facebook page my agency made – an image of his. I was a very humble, young, impressionable girl who believed in herself but was still really learning the ropes, and this comment of his almost brought me to tears of joy. It read,

"Anja Christoffersen one of those talents that occasionally pop up and "wow!" you the minute she steps in front of the camera. From the first shot to last always bubbled with unflagging enthusiasm and ideas."

I started booking in for shoots very quickly, doing an average of 3-4 shoots a week, sometimes even more.

Everyone I worked with gave me incredible feedback and told me I would achieve great things in my life. I felt as if they meant this genuinely rather than just grooming my ego. I was overjoyed they could sense my enthusiasm and passion, and were unable to tell that I was disabled as I handled myself so well.

I quickly got booked for my first ever runway, as I was blessed with good height (179cm - don't ask me what that is in feet). I *loved* my first fashion show experience. I met some great designers – some I have had the privilege of working with for years after this show in 2015.

I fell in love with runway – I would get the hugest adrenaline rush stepping onto the catwalk. All the hours walking up and down the hallway in high heels had finally paid off.

While my modelling career was taking off, I was contacted by the hospital, and told that they would be doing my surgery to divide my labia minora on Friday, ahead of my swimwear shoot the following Wednesday. My agency had organised a bonding trip to Stradbroke Island for a day that weekend. I was so excited to go and had committed to it before I knew about my surgery date. Knowing I would be out of surgery the day before I knew it was a bit too unrealistic, especially considering I would be in a bikini most of the day and would still be bleeding from the surgery.

I spoke to my manager Mary after one of the shoots I was doing that she styled and told her that I had some medical problems and had to go into surgery the day before and wouldn't be able to make the trip. Compassionately, she totally understood.

Friday came, and I fasted from Thursday midnight and had a shower at 5am, arriving at the hospital by 6am to check in for surgery as I was first on the list. I went up to the surgical suites, and was prepped – drip in, hair net, stockings and hospital gown on. My mum sat with me as I waited nervously as I had lost all conception of what it felt like to have my body cut and sewn up again with stitches.

They called me in for the surgery and I said goodbye to mum. Once wheeled into theatre, within the count of 10, I was out cold.

I woke up hazy and happy. The pain was more of a discomfort when I moved, so I was pleased. I was asked about my pain level, and scored it at a 3 – a great sign to the doctors that I was fit to be discharged. Before they would let me go I had to pee. I went to the bathroom, wobbling on my feet as I was still dizzy from the anaesthetic. I was terrified when I looked down at the pad and hospital undies filled with blood. As I peed it stung like hell and there was blood all through the toilet.

Assured by the nurses this was normal, I was fed sandwiches and cordial before being picked up by mum. As I had to be supervised after surgery, I ended up on the floor of the office once again in a little makeshift bed. I remember not telling many people what the surgery was for as I was quite shy that it was related to the appearance of my genitalia. Because of this, complaining about the pain to anyone apart from Mum was not an option for me.

By the time I got to the office and lay down. I was feeling weak and distraught. The pain had finally caught up with me after the anaesthetics and IV pain killers had worn off. Getting out of hospital was not as much of a good idea as I had thought. I didn't even have as much as Panadol with me because I thought the pain was so manageable. Boy, was I mistaken.

Mum sent one of her staff to grab me the strongest over the counter pain killer she could get her hands on. I was feeling a *bit* more relieved once I took it however it was not strong enough to make a significant difference. Every single movement with my pelvis or legs was painful, let alone the stinging when I had to pee and the amount of blood that was flowing from the wounds.

Mum took me home from work early, so I could be more comfortable. Her and I had our curiosity peaked, as she had been teasing me that when they sewed it back up they may have done a frilly edge. I certainly did not want a frilly vagina and was a bit concerned that I would now be horrified by the result of the surgery.

As my dignity had long gone out the window, mum and I got a huge mirror and sat it in between my legs to have a look at exactly what was going on down there. Despite it looking like a crime scene, I was impressed by the doctors work. No frilly edge after all.

We were planning to go up to dads that night but decided that me sitting in the car for that long would not be good for my fresh wounds, or very comfortable for me. Dad had been well the previous weekend and we had not had anything abnormal reported to us by the support staff that came in to visit him.

Mum and I called dad to let him know we wouldn't come, and he didn't pick up. Dad was usually at the surf club, hardware store or buying some groceries so we didn't stress and decided to call a bit later. We called once an hour since then, from 3pm through until 8pm, getting increasingly nervous every time. We couldn't get a hold of his neighbours to go over to see him and we were beginning to get frantic.

Mum and I decided we had to just get in the car and go up there, quickly calling once again before getting in the car, dad picked up. He didn't make his usual chirpy noises, he was breathing very heavily and there were scrambling noises like he was on the floor.

Straight away mum and I were in the car, speeding (safely) our way to dad's place.

When we got there, we found Dad in bed, bright red, with a burning fever and struggling to breathe. Dad's chest crackled in a sound mum and I knew all too well. Our immediate diagnosis was pneumonia – and we needed help. We had to call an ambulance and went straight to hospital.

When we got to the hospital, the doctors ran tests and did a chest X-Ray. The medical team told us that without medical intervention they would have expected dad to die within 8 hours. We had arrived at the hospital around 2am and we were all exhausted.

Not wanting to leave dad in emergency before we knew what the treatment plan was, I encouraged mum to go and sleep, and I would stay there. Mum refused to go home, but I managed to convince her to at least lay down and try and get a few hours rest in the car. It sounds very uncomfortable to be sleeping on the backseat of the car in a hospital parking lot, but we had some blankets and pillows in the boot to make it more comfortable. Eventually mum went off to the car and I stayed with dad.

My pain level was ridiculously high by this stage as I had not had a dose of painkillers in a while. The hospital would not give me any, even though I told them I had been in surgery that day. I went and lay in the bed next to dad, needing some relief as sitting down was so painful, and I was too weak to stand. I must have shut my eyes for ten minutes before I was barked at by a grumpy nurse to get out of dad's hospital bed. Dad and I had been sleeping soundly next to each other, and I had explained my medical situation yet this did not change the nurse's mind.

By 6:30am the doctor came to say they would take dad to the ward, so I ventured out of the hospital, waddling to keep my legs apart and not aggravate the wounds, in search on mum's car. I found it after doing a few laps around the carpark, and saw mum sleeping soundly in the back seat. I lightly knocked on the window saying "it's just me" to prevent her from getting a fright, and we both went in to dad together.

After dad spent a few days in that hospital, they still wanted to monitor his care, so they transferred him to another hospital on the Sunshine Coast where he spent a further week.

Within a week of having surgery, I had my beach shoot.

My surgical wounds weren't healed yet, despite them having stopped bleeding. I remember changing my pose and being asked to extend my body more only to wince as my fresh scars pulled and stretched.

I was very proud of myself as the photographer had no idea I had just been in surgery, or that I was in any pain. I did not want to make any excuses. I considered myself to be a professional and didn't want to let things going on in my person life (medical and with dad) to reflect in my work.

My surgery follow up appointment a few days later brought good news. The surgery had been a success and I was healing well. They found that the skin had been covering a little bit of the vaginal entrance, so without it being there I was able to move on to the third dilator, seeming like a huge leap, but in reality, it was half the size of a "functional vagina". I had a long way to go but I was over the major psychological barrier of barely progressing, as I had just been granted a leap ahead.

It was confirmed again that the urethra was inside the vagina. This meant that keeping incredibly clean was essential to infection prevention, especially when doing my dilatation.

This just made me more determined to focus on my passion rather than the illness. I felt that every step I took towards my passion, was a step further away from the illness.

I was taken aback by comments that I was living the dream. I believed I was, but really that was only portrayed by the shell of me. Those who knew of my health struggles believed that it really must not be *that* bad, or the problems were now '*fixed*' because I wore a smile throughout each struggle and seemed completely 'normal' with my clothes on.

I knew just as well my life was a combination of many experiences and facets that aren't displayed on social media or to the outside world, and the 'perfect' girls and models I was comparing myself to were only putting their best foot forward too.

I tried to think of an analogy for this, and adopted one that Alex spoke to me about - people acting as if it is the 'first date'.

Let's think about this for a moment, on the first date we don't dig up childhood trauma or tell them that we are a month late on paying our rent. We do not discuss the wart between our toes or what happens behind closed doors.

I realised that the contrast of being the incontinent girl who has to do vaginal dilatation and daily rectal washouts to what I portrayed online - the fashion model who had her hair and makeup done most days and was always gushing about the latest shoot she did. Or the reality of why I would be at the beach most weekends - not because I was privileged and wealthy and would go to my 'beach house' each weekend, but the reality of going to check up on my father who had suffered brain injury and would not move out of his coastal home.

I would compare my full self to other people's first date self. It is easy to come up short. Whether it's photos, or lifestyle, we should never assume anything about another person. We should always treat each other and ourselves with kindness as comparing ourselves to unrealistic and fabricated standards is just destructive. We will never understand the depths of another person or their perspective.

Take comfort in the fact that there will always be someone better off, and always someone worse off than you, in every facet of life.

I knew I was better off than most as I had found my passion and was following it. Things were going very well for me however it wasn't smooth sailing at all, and I was met with much criticism.

I remember I had breakfast with someone I had known since I was a child who I love and adore. They said to me, "Anja, I know you want to do modelling, but I think that it is a disgusting choice and it is one I will never support."

Most thought me pursuing modelling was a bit of a joke and didn't try to hide that they thought I would never 'make it' or do well from it. I can understand their point of view as it is a cut throat industry, but really, what isn't these days?

I booked my second runway quickly. It was for the designers graduating from a Brisbane fashion college.

I wore some stunning designs that evening and stepped into the groove more than I ever had before. I felt like I knew 100% what I was doing, had earnt my place there and *deserved* to be there. I could hold my own.

After the runway I was buzzing. I had made friends with the designers I had worked for, and initially had come to fill one designers spot and ended up walking for three. I walked out of the room where they held the runway and my arm was grabbed from the side.

Not knowing who it was, I turned to look at them and saw my mum! I had no idea she would be there! I asked her if she had seen the show, and she told me that she had decided she wanted to watch and had turned up to the event without a ticket. It so ended up that one of the people heard her asking to get in and gave her a spare ticket that they had.

I was so happy that mum had seen me, and she was gushing at how well I did, unable to believe I was her daughter – the same one that has been in and out of hospital throughout her life, and the same one that walked around the house with a double chin, bags under her eyes and a food stained singlet.

I asked mum about what outfit she liked best, and what she really thought about my walk, in comparison to the other girls that had done it many times before. I was eager to find out if there was anything I could improve on.

Mum stopped me, "wait, you walked for three designers??"

"Yes mum...." As I showed her the outfits I had worn from backstage snaps.

"OH MY GOD, I DIDN'T EVEN RECOGNISE YOU I WAS JUST LOOKING AT THE OUTFIT!!"

Thanks mum. On the positive side, she thought that I had walked well and was unable to make any critiques. She was just beaming with pride.

From mum being someone who had worn makeup once in her entire life, she became a "stage mum" (she will hate me for saying this) - continually ensuring my nails were tidy, I had no stray eyebrow hairs and that I exercise and take vitamins to maintain my physique. She would look through my photos, letting me know what I needed to be conscious of, especially pouting my lips as it seemed too sexual.

I was booking even more shoots and working with some great teams of people. I had developed a great friendship and working partnership with John, and whenever we both had free time we would come up with a shoot concept and just do it. Thanks to this I would always have updated portfolio images, and John and I could get creative and try new styles, techniques and concepts.

I knew trying to develop my career, and my portfolio, I would have to do some free work for a while. I was a lot more fortunate than some other models, who would have to pay to develop their portfolios, as I was able to do it all for free.

I began feeling frustrated that lots of the work I was doing was unpaid or worked on a barter system. Subconsciously, I felt like I "wasn't good enough" to get paid, and this would bug me non-stop. I decided to push that aside as I had only been in the industry a few months at this stage.

I decided to persist as one never quite knows what is waiting just around the corner.

XIV

Resilience

*Appreciate where you are in the moment instead of living
in the past or the future*

Becoming the model, I knew there was no room for the sick girl I could easily succumb to. I understood that if I went to a job or casting and had slumped shoulders, pale lips and was clutching my abdomen, I definitely would not get the job. I had been running at 60% health for a while now, so long that I had forgotten what 100% even felt like. I found that focusing on the moment at hand and what brought me joy, made the pain and illness fade into the background.

If I ever was considering cancelling a modelling commitment due to illness, I would think to myself, "If this was my dream modelling job would I cancel it because of how I am feeling?" Most times it was a 'no' and this stopped me from using my illness as an excuse. I had to treat each moment, no matter how significant/insignificant I judged it to be, as an important step on my path.

After each day out of the house, I would come home to bed exhausted and aching. I wasn't able to notice most of the exhaustion when I was working, it was only when I stopped.

Believing I wasn't overexerting myself, and there may be something further wrong with my health, my doctor ran further blood test. The tests uncovered I had Ross River Fever proteins in my blood and it was all traced back to those huge mosquitos I was being bitten by at the horse ranch. The timing coincided perfectly to the chain reaction of my body's decline.

My immune system was low from the stress and overworking my body through high school. I had no understanding that pushing myself so hard would influence my physical health.

My GP told me that I would experience these same systems relating to Ross River fever for years to come. Every individual's body reacts to illnesses and emotions differently. While I knew that this disease wasn't responsible for everything I was experiencing with my body, it was great to understand what was going on. I was grateful that it had not been found immediately as it meant that I had investigations with urology, bowels and gynaecology where other issues were found and treated.

Understanding what was going on with my body gave me a new take on my health and I decided that the way out of the rut I was in physically, was through my emotions and following my passion. When I was strong mentally, I felt strong physically. When I was strong physically, if I wasn't strong mentally, my physical wellbeing didn't seem to matter.

By July, John and I had submitted work to two different magazines to be published. We were overjoyed to make the cover of a local magazine and be featured in a four-page spread in an American magazine. After such a positive response to our work, John and I knew that it was the beginning of something amazing.

This boosted my confidence incredibly. It was becoming less "fake it until you make it", and more *being* 'it'.

As time flew by, castings for a regional fashion festival were upon us. This held a special place in my heart as it was in the area where my dad's place is – my only constant home over the past 15 years. The year before getting signed with my agency, I had too-ed and fro-ed about going and casting as a freelance, inexperienced model. At that time, I didn't quite have the confidence in me, or belief that I would get chosen as I was still a bit stuck in what I was told the previous year (not being able to model because of my scars).

I was never shy about my body, even when I wanted to tone up or slim down, I would still be on the beach in a bikini in a heartbeat. My scars didn't upset me, as I knew they were a part of me and my story, and even when I was told that I would not be able to show them in modelling, I was only concerned over how other people would be unaccepting of the scars.

I was always accepting of them and despite at times being curious what I would look like without them, I wouldn't wish them away for a second.

I REALLY wanted to walk in this fashion festival and was reassured that my agency believed in me as a model. If my scars *were* going to disadvantage me, I was determined to give the casting director no other reason to say no. I practiced my walk up and down the hallway more, did some great workouts leading up to it, even though my body was still quite weak, all in preparation.

I had become good friends with everyone from my modelling agency. Four of us went up in the same car together, listening to great music and having good chats the drive. We were all 'models' but felt like a bunch of laid-back girls going on a road trip.

When we arrived, makeup free and in our black bikinis (my scars on full display), we strapped our heels on and lined up ready to be called up. My heart was racing, and legs felt like jelly as I waited to walk up on the wooden pool deck at a beautiful beach resort.

I knew that self-belief was the key to my success. I needed to do my best walk, be confident and *be* the supermodel that I was dreaming of becoming.

I went up there, confident and smiling. I did my walk, said hello to the judges and I was happy with how it went. I wasn't sure if I would get the job or not, as there were three hundred other people casting, competing for approximately 30 positions. I wasn't doubting myself however was aware that there was a lot of wonderful talent around me, and I was not sure what the judges were looking for.

We were told as a group that it would take about two weeks to go through the selection process and we would be notified by email to either us or our agency.

I decided to stop thinking about it, and not be worried. I felt assured in myself that I did well, and if the energy of that fashion festival aligned with mine, then I would get the job, and if it didn't, I would just have to trust in the bigger picture that there was a reason why I would not be doing it.

The thing is we never really know what the bigger picture is, and at this stage I was discussing this extensively with Alex and listening to metaphysics lectures online about this exact topic. We always need to trust in the universe that the energy we put out is the energy we get back. We must trust that we will be able to meet our desires, and what we want, when we are happy. We need to focus on happiness and positive thoughts, believe in ourselves and know everything will come at the perfect time for us.

I knew that if I didn't book this show, even though I so desperately wanted it, that it was okay. I shouldn't judge it. If I didn't get it, it was an energy thing. If I missed out, I could be at dinner on the same night of the fashion festival and meet a casting director for a huge job overseas... you just never know why certain things happen. Whatever the outcome, I just had to trust that it was the best possible case scenario for me.

I continued with life as normal, heading to uni on the Tuesday as I was now taking a heavier subject load and needed to focus in my final trimester.

In one of the breaks in Intercultural Studies, I received a perfectly timed call on my mobile. It was a number that was unsaved on my phone, as I was so used to communicating with people over Facebook. I picked up the phone confidently, and it was David. He told me that he had just received an email from the Fashion Festival I had cast for over the weekend.

I HAD BEEN BOOKED FOR THE SHOW!!!

Everything was aligning very quickly. I was booking more shoots, being specially requested by clients, successful at castings and becoming very confident both on the runway and in front of the camera. Through focusing on what brought me joy and following my passion, I experienced an emotional shift that made me a much happier person. I no longer felt limited by seeking acceptance and pleasing others. I know that may sound crazy when working as a model, as your employment relies on other people thinking that you are "beautiful" or have the "right look", but I developed a healthy mentality that everything would work out perfectly for me.

My excitement ignited me, and I was flourishing. I developed a really positive way of looking at life and booking work as I believed that everything happened for a reason, and I should not judge it. I trusted in myself and I knew that if I didn't get a job I wanted, or the dress I wanted, or the result I wanted, that it was because there was something better out there for me, or I needed to learn something from that experience. Of course, this belief system was tested many times as I was faced with criticism and "competition", mainly imposed by others and self-comparison on social media.

I had made the transition from feeling squashed by the education system, doing what I thought would be the right thing to do to get others love and acceptance, as well as financial security and wealth for myself. I now was happy; taking a chance on myself, detached from others expectations of me and judgements of what was best for me, and was very independent in my careers, goals, mentality and aims.

I had begun directing my own shoots and had learnt a lot about personal branding and marketing myself. I gradually built a network of stylists, makeup artists, photographers and models. There was one stylist I was particularly fond of, as I just thought her work was wonderful and so well thought out. She was graduating from a creative college so was a great person to be involved with at the start of her career.

This stylist had put up a casting on Instagram looking for a model, and this other girl and I had both commented on it. This other girl was a Brisbane model too, and sweetly she must have clicked on my profile, and proceeded to follow me. This was a bit rare for people you hadn't met and models outside your agency, so I realised she must have been a sweet and supportive person. I followed her back as I was pleased to have a little connection with a kind, Brisbane model as I was sure that I would bump into her at some point.

I forgot about this and went about my daily activities. My agency encouraged me to go for a casting for another large runway company that had been around for a few years and had a great reputation in Brisbane. It was quite a large show with amazing production, so I went into it with no expectations of getting in. I just wanted to be confident and have another chance to practice and showcase my developing and improving walk.

After walking for the judges, we had to take photos in bikinis.

I took off my clothes, standing next to the other models, with perfectly toned and smooth skinned tummies, with not a single mark or blemish on them. Looking down at my own, I could see the scar from my colostomy, pull through surgery, and vesicostomy, all telling a little story about me. I found myself standing there proudly rather than holding my hands over my abdomen protectively.

Once the photos were done and we said our goodbyes to each other I carried on my day, just like any other.

Shortly after this casting, I received another much-sought confirmation from my agency that I had booked this show. Unfortunately, in the Brisbane fashion industry, and some fashion industries around the world a lot of the jobs are paid in publicity and exposure. This runway was one of those, and even though it was disheartening as exposure doesn't pay the bills or contribute to my living expenses, I was so thrilled for this opportunity.

All the selected models were invited to a compulsory runway training. I arrived at the inner city multi-level carpark, as it provided enough space for this "army of models" to practice their work and get a feel for the 50-metre length of the real runway.

I saw a girl out of the corner of my eye waving, and smiling, and I wasn't sure if I should return this notion as I had often smiled and waved at people thinking they were doing it to me, but there was someone just behind me that they were engaging with. I smiled anyway, but it was evident I was a bit confused at who it was.

At the training we were doing laps of the car park like a catwalk, focusing on the different skills in runway and ensuring all our walks were uniform and the right style for the show. After walking about 2km in my highest stilettos, I was ready to crash at home, exhausted as my immune system and body weren't as energetic as they used to be, even though I was only 17.

That night as I had my feet in a magnesium bath of fragrant Epsom salts for my muscles, I got a message from the sweet girl that I had befriended over Instagram from that stylists online casting.

"It was lovely seeing you today!" She had written. Oh dear.... I hadn't even recognised her! She was the one smiling and waving at me!!

Funnily enough, one and a half weeks later, just a few days before the big show I had been training for, I booked a shoot for a local stylist with the sweet girl from Instagram, Jasmine. We both came a bit early, and we weren't even sure if we were in the right place! We saw each other and began a wonderful conversation, clicking straight away and feeling an immediate sense of friendship, support and security.

Soon enough Jasmine and I were in our 1960s makeup and cute outfits, doing a series of images in a few different outfits. We decided we would keep in touch and do coffee sometime soon, and from that moment on a strong friendship was forged.

Fast forward a week, and I was at the runway I had been training for. This was my first huge show. I had walked many fashion shows before and was probably up to a tally of about 10-15 by this stage; fashion students graduations, private runways for designers, runways at charity events and at hotels. I was confident in my walk and ability, and just wanted my body to look great.

In preparation I tried Hot Yoga and Pilates. I got hooked and saw immediate results and sweat more than I ever have before. This probably was not the best for me as I was not re-hydrating enough, and it was putting a lot of pressure on my one kidney. Despite this, it was great for me to be lose a bit of water weight and tone up before the show.

The morning of the show, I put coconut oil through my hair to make it shiny, coated my body in black (dead) avocado I had put in the freezer for this exact purpose, and stood perfectly still without touching anything so I wouldn't get yelled at for making a mess!

I quickly jumped in the shower around 12 walked down to the show location from our apartment. My skin was glowing (I hoped after smelling like rotten avocado for the past two hours) and hair shiny. I was ready.

I walked into the huge backstage area and saw a rack with my name, photo and order number on it. I had quite a few outfits on my rack, and I was thrilled with this – it always meant for a busy, adrenaline-filled show full of quick changes and lots of runway time. I also interpreted this as an indication that I had the right look for the designers that I was walking for. This filled me with the feeling that I was accomplishing what I was told I never could.

A special designer set up in the far corner backstage. He was from overseas and very well respected, travelling to Australia specifically for the show. He was able to select his own models out of the 30 there for the show, and he would only choose about 10. I was chosen.

I went over to his corner and he put me in the most beautiful clothing, commenting that he loved my look and thought my figure was similar to Gisele's, who he had worked with previously. This was the biggest compliment ever; not sure how true it was but I loved it! I was selected to walk for him four times in the final segment.

I was thrilled for show time as Mum, Alex and my beautiful cousin's wife, were coming to watch me. This meant a lot to me as it was my biggest show to date, and I wanted them to see how far I had come - from walking up and down hallways in heels and it all being a dream, to that moment right then, backstage and ready to walk out into the flashing lights of cameras. I had earnt my place there. I even had my own dresser (so exciting!!!).

Just before line up I began feeling quite unwell. I was really dizzy. I had eaten, maybe not enough, but that was definitely not the problem as I had fasted before and been fine.

I was crouching down on the ground in my heels, unable to take them off as it was too close to show time. I had been in the same heels for the past half an hour since we began getting dressed, they were beginning to throw out my pelvis, where there is a mass of scar tissue, very sensitive to being held in a different position for a long time. My tummy began aching and my heart was racing. The nausea came first, and then the palpitations started, something that the doctors weren't able to do much about – I wasn't even nervous, I was so excited, so I knew it wasn't just a nerves thing.

I had been chronically unwell for such a long time, and it would always lure in the background to strike when I began feeling tired. I was used to functioning in short bursts of energy, but I had been holding my body so well, in and out of clothing, standing in heels, around so many people and doing a few run throughs up and down the catwalk over the past six hours. I was exhausted and my body was telling me to rest at the wrong time. I texted mum;

"I am feeling horrible but do not know what to do, I want to do the show, but my body is feeling very weak and unsteady – please ask your guardian angels to help me get through this"

I couldn't tell anyone. Being sick at a show is so unprofessional, and I would not want it to taint my reputation. I needed to handle it all internally, and as I had so many other times, smile through the pain and focus on what I wanted rather than what my body was so severely experiencing.

Regardless of my physical condition, this was my workplace and what I wanted to do for my career. I wanted nothing to stand in the way of me achieving what I set out to. So, with that spirit, the show must go on!!

XV

Acceptance

Appreciation, acceptance and love are the greatest gifts you can give to yourself and others

I was congratulated by everyone, even those that I didn't know, for how well I did at the fashion show. I had the honour of closing the show in a beautiful gown from the international designer, swishing around the midnight blue skirt of the dress as I walked. I was even more thrilled that I had this opportunity as a seventeen-year-old who had been modelling just short of 6 months.

The following weekend was the regional fashion festival, the real fulfilment of my long-term goals. The previous fortnight I had been chosen out of 10 to do a charity runway event as part of the fashion festival, so I had met the director as well as some of the other models and seen the venue. This meant I was very comfortable on show day.

When I was told in that bleak agency office that I would never be able to show my scars I never imagined that I *could* walk this coastal fashion show that was renowned for its large swimwear segment. For this reason, walking this show was symbolic. It may have been just another Saturday for some of the other models, or the cool little side thing they did once a year, but to me it was a highlight of my life.

I arrived around 8am as there was plenty to do – fittings with the designers (I was walking for about 10 different designers), rehearsals, hair, makeup and more. Some of my close friends from the agency were walking at the show too, so it was a great experience to be able to share.

As I was so serious about doing modelling as my career, I understood how valuable it was to build good relationships with the designers. As soon as I received the run sheet a month beforehand, I had researched each designer I was walking for, so I understood what the garments were like, if there was a meaning behind their work and how they started. I knew that each designer would want their clothes portrayed in a particular way, so I went out of my way to find out how I would be able to represent their brand in the way they would want.

Many of the designers there stood out for me, and I loved every one of the designers that I met and was touched in particular by three of the designers who went out of their way to have a good conversation with me. I had an amazing sense of déjà vu being there that day.

The whole energy of the fashion festival was great, everyone was bubbly, enthusiastic and kind, and I made friends with lots of members of the team.

I was riding on an all-time high that no one could knock me down from. I felt on top of the world.

I had just completed my final exams in my last trimester of my Certificate IV and was feeling relieved – also proud I had completed 'high school' in my own unique way.

For a long time, I had been wanting to go blonde as my natural blonde hair as a child had faded out into an unremarkable mousy brown. I couldn't think of a better time for a pick-me-up and decided on going blonde that weekend. New hair, new me... right?

I bought a packet mix at the chemist and attempted to do it myself (using the remainder of the mixture on my distracted mother). We both looked in the mirror. We definitely looked related at least. We also looked like we were clowns on the run from the circus, a bright orange colour coating every inch of hair on our heads.

The worst part about it was, we were going to dinner with a Danish family friend of ours, and his wife was a hairdresser – how embarrassing.

We had an emergency pit stop on the way back to Brisbane from the Coast – my cousin, who has been hairdressing since before I was born, to fix our hair. We all had a great laugh, and managed to get most of the orange out, covered by a combination of brown and blonde foils.

I loved being a blonde and was ready to adopt the mentality that blondes have more fun!!

I was booked for a shoot with a photographer the following week - my first shoot as a blonde. He had asked to shoot with me in collaboration, but I had told him that I would need to be paid and gave him my rates. It was a ballsy move as with the majority of these situations they decide to go with another model.

Since Instagram became such a widely used tool with many girls wanting to pursue modelling, photographers could find them easily and they would be willing to work for free. This meant that 'paying' in photos and exposure became legitimate as there would always be a 'model' on Instagram willing.

I was sick of being approached for free work endlessly. I was appreciative of the work but wanted to be valued. I had been booking great jobs and high-profile runways however was not making a decent income.

It was a good surprise when the photographer got back to me, happy with the rate I gave and willing to pay. I realised that I had to value myself before others would value me.

I was grateful to have a good network of friends and family around me that encouraged me to keep following what made me happy. Despite having lost contact with some of my high school friends, there were a special few that I would spend a lot of time with. It came time for them to graduate, and coincidentally I was graduating the exact same night. Even though I hadn't completed high school, I couldn't help but laugh to be graduating from my equivalency certificate IV on the same night as I would have finished high school.

It was a synchronicity you couldn't even make up. Things may not have happened in the 'easiest' way – being sick and needing to leave school to recover, however when I looked at the bigger picture I knew it worked out perfectly. If I had stayed in school, I would have never been where I was in this moment - modelling three or more times most weeks, have time to recover AND be able to excel in my studies!

There was not much fuss made around my graduation. It was just mum and I, no big dinner or afterparty. I was happy to have finished but knew it was only the beginning of my new life, so did not feel the need to celebrate hugely. Mum and I got dressed nicely and went to the campus where we had some photos taken, with me in a black graduation cap holding my certificate proudly.

At the ceremony, they handed out the certificates and transcripts to each of us. They then proceeded to give academic awards for high achievement. Throughout my studies I had received mid-semester awards for five subjects. I had my hopes up that I would receive something however had no expectation.

When reading through the names, they had only four students from our campus that received awards. I was one of them! Confidently I strode forward and collected my award as mum beamed with pride.

When I came back I tugged at mum's arm, "Let's go, it is all over now!"

"No Anja, just wait until the ceremony is finished!" Mum responded.

I was just hungry and hoping for some celebratory fast food on the way home.

The MC began explaining the DUX award, for the student with the highest-grade point average. We were told it was the highest-achieving student across both campuses, selected from at least 200 or more students. I had no gauge of others results, especially those students at the other campus.

I had almost convinced mum to make a run for it when the announcer read out my name, followed by "DUX".

WOW. This was my dream – as dorky as that sounds! It was the cherry on the cake. I realised them that I really could have both – academic success and follow my modelling dream.

I had easily gained entry into the Nursing program and had already been given an Offer of Place, as well as into Business at another university. Considering nursing, I understood that working with ill people when I had a low immune system was not appropriate. Mum encouraged me to pursue business, as I had a good business brain and achieved very, very highly in my marketing subject.

I reviewed the safe option (uni) and the risky option (going out on my own and following my passion with modelling). I usually wasn't a HUGE risk-taker, so making the decision to pursue modelling felt as if I had jumped off a platform and was flapping my wings without a safety blanket. It wasn't a bludge decision, it was the decision to follow my heart.

I had always pictured myself going to University, ever since I was that little baby getting pushed around her pram, looking up at the pictures of the different universities and dreaming big dreams.

I stopped understanding the point of having a certificate saying I knew something. I wanted to learn by life experience, something I felt I would be sheltered from stuck in classrooms and lectures for the next three or more years. The career I wanted wasn't something a degree could give me. It was a career on the international stage as a model and advocate that anything is possible despite the body or circumstances you are born into.

Something my mother said when I was young had always stuck with me…

"If only when you were a baby, in and out of hospital, or when I had first found out the diagnosis, I could have seen you now. It would have saved me so many tears, and so much heartache, because I would have known there was hope for my little baby, and that she could still live a good life."

I wanted to be more than just a model. I wanted to be a role model. I wanted to walk on the international catwalks on my own merits, not have it gifted to me as the token ambassador disabled girl. I wanted to make it myself, so I could say that I did it. I wanted to inspire people with my condition and any rare disease or chronic illness that they could follow their dreams regardless of their diagnosis. I wanted to bring hope to the mothers of sick babies that they can get through it and flourish. I wanted to be the positive success story that empowers others to follow their joy and passion, no matter what it is, and no matter the odds that are against them.

I knew walking fashion shows in Brisbane wasn't a high enough target. I had to set my sights on something bigger.

I knew whatever energy I put out, I would get back. I knew that my reality was created by the emotions that I feel, the thoughts that I think and the beliefs that I fuel. I knew whatever I focused on expanded – positive or negative. I was determined I could do it.

So, I did.

It was the festive season of 2015. We had our traditional Danish family Christmas on Christmas Eve, where my cousin confided in me that she was expecting her second child. We had developed a close friendship and it was such a joy to find out about her pregnancy as she had struggled with conceiving in the past. I knew this baby would be very special because of how much it was wanted, and how much it was already loved.

Still on a high from the roast pork and gravy, I set off to Sydney on Christmas Day to meet Alex down there as planned. We were spending New Year's Eve on the huge balcony of a penthouse apartment looking over the Sydney harbour and watching the fireworks with some of her friends. When I say huge, I really mean HUGE. You could fit a two-bedroom apartment in the space of this balcony.

Alex had given me a stunning floor length black dress, with a cowl neck and delicate white beading in an intricate pattern at the top of the dress before fading out to nothing as you moved further down. It had a beautiful open back with just a string tied, holding the sides in. It fell beautifully, lightly grazing my figure before falling to the ground.

I did my hair up in a tight low bun and coated my lips with a bright red lipstick.

The night was a blur of flowing champagne, city lights, exquisite fireworks with loud crackles and bangs, glowing balloons and lots of laughter.

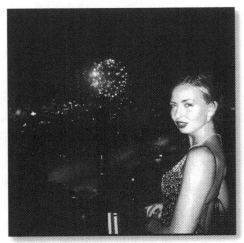

New Year's Eve 2015

After midnight, once the firework show had concluded, we were ready to head home as it had become quite cold and blustery.

When we arrived at the house where we were staying, I took off my makeup and slipped into bed with my notepad and a pen. I had a tradition of setting some new year goals and was scribbling them down as my mind drifted away with my imaginings. I desperately wanted them to come true, and I knew I had to believe they could happen if I ever wanted to have chance of living them.

Written in cursive on the blank page; 1. get more Bridal work, 2. travel interstate and internationally for modelling and 3. walk in an official fashion week overseas. Satisfied with my decision, I closed my eyes as I practiced my visualisation of all of these coming true.

2016 was going to be the year of achieving my dreams.

XVI

⋘∞⋙

Determination

The first step to achieving your goals is believing you will

I was determined. I would follow my joy with wholehearted belief. I knew these were big goals for a relatively new model in the industry, especially one from Brisbane signed with a boutique modelling agency. What is the point of setting easy goals *anyway*?

Alex and I flew out of Sydney on the second of January. That same day I was booked for a Bridal Expo on the fifth at one of the best Wedding Venues in Queensland.

A few days after landing, I was at the wedding venue, getting my makeup and hair done beautifully, being adorned with an exquisite floral crown and bouquet and able to wear two different wedding gowns by a talented Sunshine Coast bridal designer. One was a princess type style with a beaded bodice, satin waistband and tulle skirt. The other was this cute white shorts playsuit with a tie up cowl neck, and a wraparound chiffon skirt, that could be added or removed.

We did two beautiful fashion shows throughout the day and I was then interviewed on the news and asked to do a few twirls in the dresses!

I got beautiful photos and made a lot of great contacts and friends at the event. One of the photos was published in a popular print Bridal magazine shortly after. I had ticked off the first goal of the year and it was still only the first week of January!

Amazing synchronicities began happening - a designer from a fashion festival I walked for, had linked up with David, as he captured some great images of her designs on the catwalk. Coincidentally they were the only ones she had as the official photographer had experienced a technical failure. As I had interacted so well with her, she asked if she could hire both me and David to shoot the cover for a local lifestyle magazine with a 40,000-copy circulation as she had been contracted on as the stylist and fashion editor.

I shot that in January ahead of a February cover, and had my hair and makeup done by one of the makeup artists I had become good friends with. I was in such a happy and comfortable environment and was having such a wonderful time. The pictures were great, and it made for the perfect cover when it came out – I could barely believe it was me! I had really stepped into the persona of the model.

Everything was just flowing, and I was beginning to get a lot of bookings for different runways and shoots, rather than being put forward in a group and being selected that way.

My modelling agency got a contract with a large online clothing retailer to take photos for their website. They got to choose from the models in the agency and chose me for their first shoot.

I woke up early for the shoot that was to be held at a public pool. I was up at 5am to do my makeup and at the shoot by 6am, to catch the morning light and be there before it got busy and crowded. I had begun doing a bit of work here and there with my family business and had an agent conference to attend at one of the universities shortly after. The timing would work perfectly as the uni was in walking distance from the shoot location.

We were shooting swimwear, so I put each of the ten swimwear outfits on and began posing. These photos were beautiful, the light was soft, and the background was magical. The shoot went so quickly, I was in the zone and feeling really happy with my body. The photos looked wonderful and I could not wait to see them on the website.

I went and got changed into corporate clothes, and walked myself over to the agent's function, getting there 15 minutes early. Everyone at the function knew me well as Riborg's daughter, as she is a celebrity in the education agent industry. I glided through the presentations easily and in the activities we did I was getting all the answers right, just off my basis of knowledge growing up in the business and listening to the presentations.

I was progressing very well as a model; my posing had improved and I was able to move fluidly from pose to pose. It just came very naturally to me. I was always presented perfectly and in a happy, confident mood and spoke eloquently. This dedication as well as being able to engage other people easily, landed me another great opportunity that I had not even realised existed before.

Ever since I was standing on top of the table at the age of two, making speeches at family gatherings, I have always wanted to speak in front of large audiences. I was right in my comfort zone when David asked me to join him in a presentation for a large photography group to discuss modelling photography.

I did not plan a speech, as David told me that he would just direct me to demonstrate simple poses and throw in a few words where necessary.

It turned out almost half the presentation was me speaking, sharing my opinion about fashion photography and other tips and tricks on posing models, making them feel comfortable and engaging with them so the photos turn out even better!

I loved this experience and did not get stumped for words once. I spoke very clearly, and shared insights I didn't even realise I had.

In the days to follow, David said he had raving reviews from the photography group and could not have been happier by the presentation we did together. I knew this was opening a great door for my future in terms of speaking in front of audiences, I was just unsure of what form it would take at this stage.

I began working out again more at the gym to improve my health, immune system and get more toning. I was going every day to every second day, doing workouts a lot less strenuous to my plan the previous year as I was focused on building my body to be strong and resilient rather than appearance oriented.

Jobs were booking left, right and centre, and I really was modelling 'full time'. I was really glad I had made the decision to follow my excitement rather than go to university as if I had I would not have been able to accept all the opportunities that had been offered to me.

By Mid-March, I was cover for the second time for the same online magazine and was featured inside in a four-page spread interview with more photos. All photos were taken by my manager Mary, who had a hidden talent for photography. As we loved each other as people, we got on really well as a team and produced some amazing shots.

After a few more shoots, I was off to Sydney to look after my God sister's three kids while she went away with her partner. I was so excited at this opportunity as I loved her kids and could have a little holiday in Sydney.

I had the smallest taste of being a 'mother' – having to cook, clean up and keep coming up with fun things to do. While I was having a wonderful time, I was also quite exhausted.

I loved the concept of house sitting and looking after kids and was beginning to think of this as an opportunity to subsidise my modelling income.

While I was down in Sydney I got a call from mum, "Hey Anja, Alex and I are going to Amsterdam, do you want to come?"

OF COURSE, I WANTED TO COME!! "Why are you going to Amsterdam mum?" I asked.

"I really want to go to a Conference being held there!" she explained, with excitement in her voice.

Alex and I had always joked of going to Amsterdam for my eighteenth birthday, and this would only be two months before it. It was always our little plan and fun visualisation that we never gave deep thought to. Out of the blue, mum was making it happen!

On my return home from Sydney, I was invited by my manager to come and train some of the newer models in runway. I had been working so hard on my runway walk since I was fourteen and this just reconsolidated that my hard work had paid off.

It was a warm, sunny day on the rooftop of one of the inner-city carparks, with scenic 360-degree views of Brisbane. A strong, cooling breeze soothed the burn of our sun kissed skin.

There were only two girls at this training as it was quite low-key, and focused on developing basic runway skills as both girls had no experience.

I was able to train these two girls individually while Mary shot with the other one.

I was taught runway but had never been taught to teach. Most of my runway skills were developed in the hallways in my own home after watching fashion week videos and Victoria's secret on loop.

I began by aligning the girls' posture, getting their body stretched tall, hips aligned and shoulders back before beginning on how to walk. I would get them to walk to the best of their ability first, before adding on skills to focus on one by one.

It was a special feeling seeing the improvement in both girls from their first walk to when we finished the session. I knew in this moment that it would be something that I would love to do more of in the future.

Another day, another shoot… and this next one was another with Jasmine!

On shoot day, Jasmine and I were jolted awake by the alarm, pulling on our clothes and heading there.

The photographer, Jasmine and I arrived simultaneously at the shoot location, as we got out of the car carrying big garment bags of the clothes we sourced. As we went inside Jasmine and I were thrilled to both see familiar faces of makeup and hair stylists we had worked with previously.

We got our hair and makeup done, beginning with a simpler, natural look to compliment the stunning pieces I had borrowed from the designer I was shooting with in two days' time.

As the shoot progressed, Jasmine and I both began to feel quite unwell. Most of the time I wasn't feeling too well and was used to running at under 100% however it was beginning to take its toll. We had both been up early and hadn't had the chance, or been responsible enough to have breakfast, as we didn't feel like eating so early, or want our stomachs bloated for the shoot.

I hadn't been eating very much lately as I did not have enough energy to keep up my exercise routine and did not want that to impact on my body and for me to gain weight. I was in an industry where anorexia was fashionable, and I felt as if I could not afford to become much heavier, despite being an AU size 6.

I really was not well, however Jasmine wasn't feeling good either, so I questioned if it was just something in the air or something we had eaten the previous day.

I remember constantly looking out for Jasmine as I knew that she was feeling a bit faint, however neither of us wanted to compromise our professionalism by telling anyone on set. If I could see her begin flailing I would ensure that she sat down and had some water as I knew the feeling of being unable to rely on your body when you were trying to work.

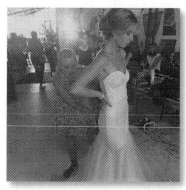

Behind the Scenes at the shoot

We were in the fifth hour of a shoot that was supposed to be three hours. I wouldn't have cut a second short, but it was becoming difficult to keep myself up right and I had a lot of pain in my back. It was very common for me to have pain in my back when wearing very high heels for a long time, so I had dismissed it as nothing. What was becoming difficult to control was my racing heart, exhaustion in my body and dizziness. I was working overtime keeping it masked so no one could tell that I was unwell.

By the time we left it was about 4:30pm, and we had been at the shoot since 8:30am from memory. We had taken our time packing up as we were both trying to wind down after the shoot. On the way home, we went through a fast food drive through (our little secret) to try and restore all the calories we had burnt!

As soon as I got home I crawled into bed, completely exhausted and feeling very weak.

I slept in in the morning, and when I woke up mum had already left for work. I was still feeling horrible but thought a day of rest in bed would ensure I was ready for my big campaign shoot the following morning.

When the clock chimed 10am, the discomfort in my back was increasing, until it became an incredibly overwhelming cramping pain. Even with my high pain threshold, I was in tears and my voice was shaking. I called mum to tell her what I was experiencing and ask for her medical advice. She asked me about the pain, and after pinpointing it was more on the left side (where my only kidney is), she raced me straight to the doctors.

I have been going to the same GP and medical practice since I was born. As they understand my medical condition, if I ever have to see a doctor immediately, they just rejuggle things to fit me in. I called them on the way in the car and they notified my doctor and ensured I could be seen straight away.

Within seconds of describing my pain to my GP, a referral letter was written, and I was on the doorstep of the emergency department at the hospital. They took me straight in and ran blood and urine tests as well as scans.

It was always incredibly difficult to pinpoint the need to check for a UTI as I have never had any stinging when peeing as I don't have the nerves! This meant it could be ruled out incorrectly if I was just asked about the sensation when I peed.

Just as my GP had predicted, I had a severe kidney infection. I felt horrible. I had been unwell for days but was in denial as I had been feeling so alive planning for the upcoming shoots and so dedicated that I hadn't wanted to cancel them just to stay in bed and rest all day.

I was moved to the ward where I was having strong antibiotics pumped into my veins to try and stop the infection in its tracks. My kidney being my only one, meant infections had to be taken very seriously, especially with the ultrasound showing swelling and fluid in and around my kidney.

By the time it was 7pm, the doctors were due to do their nightly round on the ward. Mum and I conspired to try and get them to let me go home. Mum's intentions were focused on being able to get a good night's sleep at home, whereas mine were more centred around my shoot in the morning.

Sure enough, with a smile and insisting I felt strong, great and pain free (lie), I was allowed to go home with antibiotics and painkillers, as well as strict instructions to return if my condition worsened.

In an effort to stay professional, I did not cancel my shoot as it was an opportunity I did not want to miss and knew it would be horrible to leave the designer in the lurch.

At 6:30am I was picked up by my friend who I was modelling with for this shoot and drove an hour to Bribie Island. I was feeling completely out of it, but the hospital had given me stronger painkillers, so I took a pill and my antibiotics, and just let my body feel relief. I was second into hair and makeup so was able to sit down for the first one and a half hours, apart from helping carry a few things down onto the beach.

Walking along the sand carrying things was so difficult for my frail body. Every step, heartbeat and breath were an effort for me by that stage.

As soon as I got my makeup on, I was well into the persona of the model. I was able to shoot very quickly, only 5-10 minutes per look. Being able to work in short energy bursts was easier for me, as when I started to feel exhausted I could have a tiny break while my friend was shooting.

We worked very effectively, meaning by 1pm we were able to pack up and head home again. Apart from telling the team my previous day's adventures, there weren't even able to tell I was unwell.

As soon as I got home I crawled into the comfort of bed once again, painkillers and antibiotics within reach. I was just exhausted.

I was so passionate, that I did not give the illness a chance to force me into giving up something I loved. I thought if I was able to ignore the feeling of illness long enough and only focus on the joy I got from what I was doing; I would transform into being healthy. At the risk of seeming hypocritical as I was only just out of hospital, what I was doing was working well for me so far. I was a lot stronger than I had been 1 year ago.

I whisked myself out of bed before midday the day following my shoot and caught a bus into the city for another runway training Mary had invited me to instruct. I was so excited at this prospect that there wasn't a chance in hell that I would cancel it just because of a kidney infection. I thought to myself, "As long as I could stand, I was well enough to keep going".

This went on for days, working day after day - training models, shooting, going to events and giving another presentation. All of this while recovering from my infection. I was trying to fit in as much work as possible before heading over to Europe.

It was only a fortnight before my flight. I was going to Denmark for a week to see my sister and her family, before meeting mum and Alex in Amsterdam.

As my dream was to model in Europe, and walk in a fashion week there, I tried to google some agencies online that were open to international models. I found an open casting for one in Denmark and sent my digitals (no makeup photos) and a black and white headshot from one of my beach shoots with John to an International mother agency in Amsterdam.

I had done my part; the rest was in the hands of the universe!

XVII

International

It is not the places you travel that will amaze you, but the opportunities that travel presents you with – to expand your view of the world and understanding of yourself

After stress of last minute packing and the latest candidate for a random bomb test and security pat down, I was at the International airport about to hop on a plane to Denmark, via Dubai and Schiphol (Amsterdam) airport.

I could not wait to spend time with my sister and her family once again and meet Alex and mum in Amsterdam. I was equally excited as I had received a reply from the modelling agency in Amsterdam, and we had arranged to meet on the second day of my trip for a casting to get into the agency.

Landing in Denmark was breathtaking. Last time when I had been it was dark, rainy and cold - so to be there in May when the sun is shining bright, all the trees have fresh leaves and the flowers blooming was a huge contrast.

We had dinner in the beaming 7pm rays of the European summer sun out in my sister's garden. We enjoyed a spread of delicious Danish meats, sauces, salads and more while having long-awaited quality time together. It the perfect greeting to Copenhagen.

It was my first Danish summer since I was a child. I had forgotten how many hours of light there was. I was blown away when I went to bed at 10pm and it was still light outside, barely showing signs of the sun beginning to set.

The weather was an idyllic 18 degrees Celsius and could jump up to as high as 24. My sister and I were inseparable as we recognised that the week that we were spending together would not be anywhere near enough time.

On the third day, after picking up the boys (my nephews) from school, we went home and changed, ready to catch the metro into the city, and go to Tivoli. While we were in the city I was going to call into the modelling agency there and introduce myself. The worst they could say was 'no'.

I put on my tight black singlet, tight black jeans and boots, with my thin stilettoes in my hand to change into before walking in. We walked through the city as people sat out in the sun at cafes and rode their bikes up and down the narrow streets. Finally, we got to the modelling agency. I leant on the wall while I strapped on my shoes and strode inside as my sister and the boys waited in the cobblestone street for me.

I walked in through the big glass doors and introduced myself. I was asked to fill in an application form with all my details. They told me they usually did not represent people who are based in other countries, especially outside of Europe, but they would consider me. They led me in to another room, styling props lining one wall and a white studio background lining the other, opposite large windows that looked over a small courtyard. They asked me to stand in basic poses and took a series of photos of me at every angle. I said a warm goodbye as I left their office and returned down to my sister.

I felt really happy with how it went, and my sister was excited at the prospect that I could be spending more time in Denmark with her. I took a few photos in the street, holding my portfolio book and feeling so accomplished. I would never have been confident enough to do that just a few years earlier.

I changed into my sensible shoes, as we weaved our way through the streets to Tivoli. Tivoli is the second oldest theme park in the world, and the second most popular seasonal theme park globally, as it is only open in select months each year. I had been briefly in my trip to Denmark when I was 15 but was very excited to explore it during late spring nights.

As we walked in we were greeted by live concerts and music at every turn, beautiful lanterns lining the paths and gardens filled with blooming tulips. It made all Australian theme parks look cheap to say the least. This was on a whole new level.

My sister and I were both matching in all black, now with the addition of black coats and aviator sunglasses as the temperature began to drop.

I went with my nephews on a few rides, the eldest and I going on the "scariest" ride at the theme park.

We were tightly strapped into our seats on this ride called Vertigo which had a g-force level of 5. Like most carnival rides designed for an adrenaline rush, you were flung through the air, twisting and turning in every direction, switching between upside down and right way up before you could even realise what was happening.

We had a beautiful dinner looking over the canal in Tivoli, before enjoying some live music, until it was after 9pm (but still light)!

The rest of the time in Denmark flew by. We went for long walks, explored all the touristy spots as I never get tired of them, and saw the Copenhagen football team win the Championship.

With a sad farewell, I got on a plane back to Amsterdam, anticipating seeing my mum and Alex, and having our first international holiday all together.

When I arrived, I looked at the map of Schiphol airport sent by my usually disorganised mother and found the meeting spot where we had agreed to find each other. I found my way to the spot quite easily, standing there and triple checking it was the right place. They were scheduled to arrive half an hour before me, so I was concerned not to find them there waiting for me. I couldn't phone or message them, as mum is the least reliable person with her retro Nokia mobile phone.

I was waiting there with my bags, twiddling my thumbs. I kept checking the board and monitoring their flight, that had landed on time and the baggage claim was closing. I waited and waited, until the flight disappeared off the board altogether. I knew Alex was unwell and I was concerned that something had happened in transit and nothing had been communicated to me.

I left the meeting spot and wandered up and down the airport looking for them. I searched and searched, and they were nowhere to be found. I went back to the original meeting place with faith they would turn up there eventually.

After another 15 minutes had passed, I was just about to lose all hope when I see two blonde ladies hurrying across the airport side by side, laughing. That was them. Thank god they were here!

They didn't seem to have an explanation for the timing, however Alex explained to me the traumatic flight that involved my mother spilling her drinks down Alex's crotch three consecutive times. This gave us all a great laugh as we wandered out into the cool spring air and jumped in a taxi.

We were staying in the heart of Amsterdam, off one the *million* canals.

After dropping our bags off, Mum and I ventured out into the cobblestone streets in search of a grocery store. Europe is just a whole different energy than Australia, and it felt like a movie as I walked past deli's, extravagant bakeries and artisan shops. We wandered through and found a grocery store and were amazed at the variety and assortment of foods. We picked up a few basic groceries and carried them back to the apartment.

As Mum and Alex both went to have an afternoon nap, I put on my exercise clothes and running shoes, as I needed to let off some steam from a boy problem and tone up ahead of my casting the following day.

I left a note and took a key card, leaving my phone in the apartment. I did not have any phone reception or an international sim card, and mum confessed that she had left her phone at home, so I trusted I would be just as safe without it.

I rarely run these days, and if I ever do it means that I am feeling *very* overwhelmed. I did not know where to go, but just kept running. I started by heading along from our apartment, down the streets, across bridges with canals flowing underneath, through little lanes and around the more residential area of inner city Amsterdam.

I did a big loop, about a 3km run and barely stopped to walk once which is unheard of for me. My energy was flowing, and I had a lot more clarity than before. I went back to the apartment and the key card would not work, I could not get it to open the door no matter what I tried. I was banging on the door for mum or Alex to come and get me, but they mustn't have heard as it did not warrant any response.

I thought I should just go for a while more until I knew they had been able to get enough rest. I went back downstairs and wondered in to the city centre, with other tourists stopping me for directions as I was being confused as Dutch. I wouldn't be of any help, and the other tourist and I just laughed as I said that they would have to ask a local.

I walked further and further through the city, trying my best to remember the way back and jokingly thinking to myself that I should have left a trail of breadcrumbs. I was overcome by the beauty of Amsterdam, it was filled with so much culture, more people riding their bikes than I had ever seen before, and heritage terrace houses lining the intricate geometry of the canals.

I must have been 'exploring' for close to two hours, just taking in all of the scenery before deciding to return back to the apartment as I could feel it was getting late.

This time when I knocked on the door mum opened it, happy to see me.

We decided to have a relaxed night in, and mum and I ventured out to get takeaway Indian food, an unusual first meal to have on arrival in Europe.

After we had dinner, the boy problem intensified and he made a threat.

It was 11pm at night and I really needed to get some rest. I had no idea what to do in the situation I was in. I stood in the shower, eyes red and puffy, tears streaming down my face, my breathing ragged and heart racing.

Tomorrow was my big day with the casting. Tomorrow quickly became today as it reached into the early hours of the morning as I slipped into bed to try and get some sleep.

I woke up at 2:30am, only having had two hours sleep, and wandered towards the light into the lounge room, where I found mum and Alex sitting and drinking tea. I was still so upset and they could read it off me. Without it having to be spoken, we all agreed that if I felt this way in the morning, there was no way I was going to pull off the casting and have a chance at fulfilling my goal.

It was a lot of pressure on my shoulders. I understood energy. The things I wanted would be drawn to me when I was happy, and in alignment with them, and if I was still wearing sadness on my shoulders I would only attract things of the same feeling. By feeling so upset, I knew I was just pushing away the good things that were waiting for me.

We discussed the situation with the boy more between us, Alex and mum encouraging me to just let it go. They told me that he was lying about loving me, as if he really did feel that way, he would have never put me in the position he did.

When I cry, my eyes puff up like you've never seen before. I look like tweety bird – three quarters eyelid, one quarter eye. I did not know much about the European fashion industry, but what I did know was that there were not looking for a Looney Tunes cartoon.

Alex and mum comforted me through the night - they put some of their used teabags in the freezer for my eyes in the morning, some castor oil on my face and stroked my hair back as I fell asleep on the sofa, with the sun rising over the canal pouring light into the apartment.

By the time it got to 6:30am there was no chance of me being able to sleep any longer. I got up, left on the sofa alone as Alex and mum had long since gone to bed. I went and grabbed the teabags from the freezer and pat them onto my eyes, trying to avoid getting a complete brain freeze.

I had to be at my casting by 1pm, but Alex had a gut feeling about us getting there long ahead of time, as she felt that there may be an issue with the traffic or something preventing us from going. I stood there looking at myself in the mirror - the castor oil having left my hair in oily clumps framing my face and my eyes still red, in the process of deflating back to their normal size. The great thing about a good cry is it usually makes my lips plump up. I had to work hard to find that positive.

I had made it this far and I was determined not to let last night's altercation, impact on today's happiness. I chose then and there that I was going to have good day.

I brought out my makeup bag and kissed my face with a touch of lip liner and eyeliner mixed together on my cheeks, eyelids and lips. It gave me a healthy glow – the 'no makeup' makeup look. I put on my same black singlet and tight jeans however something was pushing me to wear something slightly different. I slipped on my black woollen turtle-neck top - giving a very European look. I put on my big black boots and coat, heading out into the brunt of the sprinkling rain with mum and Alex.

We went further into the city, finding a sweet, small cafe, in the hustle and bustle of bikes whizzing past and hungover men scavenging for food after a big night out. We ordered teas and coffees, two croissants to share between us and a plate of roughly sliced Dutch cheese. We broke the bread between us, sipping our hot drinks and laughing, while the rain drizzled down in the background.

Once we had finished our breakfast, we stepped out into the cold and headed for the most convenient area for a taxi to pick us up and take us to the hotel where the casting was being held.

We arrived there so early, so we went into the back-glasshouse area of the hotel while mum got gin and tonics for her and Alex, and I tried to get in the zone for the casting, butterflies of nerves and anticipation fluttering in my stomach. I chose not to drink anything.

I didn't really feel like I 'had it' at that stage. My heart was still aching from last night and it had rippled through my body causing me to feel quite uneasy.

I wanted to be signed with this agency in the Netherlands more than anything. If I had a fairy godmother at that point in time, it is what I would have asked for. Modelling was my dream, passion and profession. I had been training for the last year, and I wanted to run in the big leagues now.

Mum brought out her and Alex's gin and tonics. I slipped off into the hotel bathroom, patting down the back of my neck with a paper towel dampened by some lukewarm water. I threw the paper in the bin and looked my reflection right in the eyes. I have never really used the athlete self-talk before a big game, or the motivational speaking on myself like you see on the Nike commercials with the likes of Michael Jordan and Tiger Woods.

I thought now was a better time than ever to try it. If it worked for these guys, it should work for me.

"Anja, come on, snap out of it... you are ready for this... you have been working for this... you deserve this... you *are* the International model, you *are* the Supermodel... now pull your sh*t together and start acting like it"

I threw my head back massaging my scalp to add some volume to my glossy hair that had fallen flat on my crown. I gave myself a determined, fierce look in the mirror, before turning into a sweet smile and a wink. I strode back out to the girls, confidently, one foot in front of the other doing my model walk. Now, I've got this.

Mum was still playing with the black cocktail stirrer trying to fish out a black speck from her drink while Alex watched on in amusement. Crying out, "have I got it?! Have I got it?!" as mum squinted her eyes, trying to find the black speck on her black utensil, we could only help but laugh. Once we assured mum it was no longer in her drink, she began smashing the life out of this thin cucumber peel, mixing the flavour into her drink.

I began filming as I knew this would end up as a good Amsterdam memory. Mum takes a sip of the drink and scrunches up her face, questioning why it tasted so strongly of cucumber and complaining she did not like the taste.

Alex offered mum her drink, mum immediately declining, insisting it would taste like cucumber too.

"That's because you have been hitting yours!!" Alex exclaimed. It was like watching a cartoon inching closer to a climax.

Mum nodded, reaching over for Alex's drink to taste, downing the first mouthful while Alex opened her mouth to say, "That is pure gin you dick!!! I haven't poured the tonic in it yet!!"

"OOOOOOOOOOOOGHHHH" Mum moaned, hand coming straight to her mouth as her face curled up into a mass of lines while her head involuntarily shook. HAHAHAHAHAHAHHAHAHAHAH!!!

All caught on video, I saved it for later. It was SOOOO funny.

It came time that I was due to meet with the modelling agency. I left the girls giggling and strode into the lobby of the hotel, eyes scouring the room in search of any indication that the people wondering around the reception area and restaurant were from the modelling agency.

I sat down on one of the sofas, grasping my portfolio in one hand, legs crossed and back stretched as tall and straight as it possibly could be.

I kept checking the time on my pone, it was just after the arranged meeting time and I could not see them anywhere. I got up and went and asked mum and Alex their thoughts, and they told me I should go back and wait, ask reception and approach anyone who looked like they could be there for the same casting.

I went and asked the lady at reception and she told me that unfortunately she knew nothing about it. I sat back in the same position on the sofa, my eyes working overtime searching for some clue.

Just when I was about to give up, I saw a tall, slender girl with chocolate brown hair and eye-catching features, walk into the hotel with her mother. They resumed a similar search to me, and I knew that I would have a friend.

I walked over to her. "Excuse me, are you here for the modelling casting?"

"Yes, I am!" she said, looking incredibly relieved to have found me. She was with her mother, who was absolutely stunning.

We both looked together for the modelling agent however could not find them, so we decided to send them a message, and go sit in the restaurant and wait for a response. Conversation began flowing, and I found out that she had driven over from Germany and had been doing quite a lot of modelling over there, and now wanted representation in the Netherlands.

We forgot about the time, and just kept talking on and on. We were interrupted by a lady, asking if we were here for the modelling casting. They were sitting at the table right next to ours conducting interviews. We both said yes and gave them our names. They said mine was not on the list, and after checking on their emails they saw that they had forgotten to add it after sending me confirmation of the meeting time.

They asked who wanted to go first, and the other girl and her mother insisted I went first, as they knew I had been at the hotel since mid-morning, and it was now mid-afternoon.

I sat down across from two ladies. There was a huge glass panel behind them, extending meters above their heads and looking out into a thin layer of fine birch trees. I introduced myself, telling them that I was from

Australia and handing my book and comp card over to them. They scanned both quickly and commented that I have a lot of swimwear content before realising that it being an Australian portfolio made it very understandable. They looked a bit sceptical, explaining the industry in Europe was much more focused on the fashion side of things, and I would have to develop that aspect of my portfolio and work on a few different things with my expressions.

They asked if I had done much runway, and I said yes. Wanting to see footage, I whipped out my phone (connected to wifi) and searched YouTube for one of the fashion shows I walked, scrolling through the video clip until it got to my part. They watched and nodded as my heart raced and I tried to read them.

We began discussing my motives, how long I had been modelling and why I was interested in modelling in the Netherlands and being represented by them. They told me that they were an International mother agency, and they did not usually pay for models to fly over to Amsterdam and provide accommodation, however they did arrange international placements with modelling agencies around the globe. We worked on the hypothetical of me being signed with them, and how it would work. They told me that as long as I was in Amsterdam they could get me work and could also place me elsewhere internationally, just could not fund my stay there.

I told them I understood completely and was not fazed by it. I said I was more than happy to pay my way in an effort to extend my career internationally. At that moment, I was exuberant, glowing with an energy of anticipation.

I was taken away near the stairwell to get my measurements and some digitals done. They were very happy with how I moved in front of the camera, even for the digitals, and my measurements were good as well.

I went back to the modelling agency director and she saw the photos and measurements and asked my how long I was in Amsterdam for. "Only ten days, that's a shame... Fashion week castings are just coming up and the shows are in early July" she told me.

I said that Fashion Week was very important to me, and if they thought it would be worthwhile I was more than happy to extend my trip and have an open-ended ticket and see what happened with fashion week castings. This left a big smile on all our faces, and they said they would love to represent me in the Netherlands and would be in contact within the next week.

OMG OMG OMG OMG OMG!!!

I raced out to mum and Alex. "I DID IT!!! I ACTUALLY DID IT!! THEY SAID THEY ARE GOING TO TAKE ME!!"

I will never forget the moment; it was like it was in slow motion. My mum reached out and gave me a big hug, tears welling up in her eyes - a mixture of pride and being worried she was going to lose her little girl to Europe.

We left the hotel much happier than we were when we came in, getting in a big black van taxi as I waved goodbye to the people from the modelling agency and said thank you.

Mum and Alex could not stop gushing that this was the beginning of my new life. They told me that the opportunity was now, and I should not miss it, and they suggested that I cancel my flight and stay in Amsterdam and ride the wave.

I was more than a little hesitant at the thought of being left in a foreign country alone. I mean really by myself, the cub out in the wild, all "ALONE"?

"Okay Anja, this is actually what you wanted. It's your goal. Do it." was my self-talk.

This was a big opportunity for me, and it would be too much of a shame if I was too scared to take it.

XVIII

⟨∞⟩

Amsterdam

Go into every situation with an open heart and an open mind

Mum's first love was a Dutch man, a student doctor who swept her off her feet and played the guitar. They had got back in contact after many, many years only recently - when he came to Australia for a holiday with his wife of 40 years. Mum had invited them both to come with us to the conference – the sole reason we were all in Amsterdam in the first place. They were coming to pick us up, so we could all go together.

We were all getting ready in the morning, mum incredibly giggly in anticipation of seeing him once again, as well as all the men that she had been watching on YouTube for the past year.

Alex and I were incredibly amused by all mum's excitement. I had already met mums first love (MFL) when he was in Australia but was eager for Alex to meet him as well.

Right on schedule, him and his wife picked us up from our apartment and we drove into a countryside looking area to a large conference centre. The Dutch man running the conference had been exchanging emails with mum, after mum wrote to him, "Why did I see you in my coffee cup?" after seeing some coffee grains resembling a photo of him at the beginning of the year. I was amused mum had written such a strange message to an absolute stranger who had thousands of people watching his videos.

I was not sure what to expect from the conference, despite

understanding most, if not all of the concepts that were on the agenda for the day's program. The day was a blur of sitting in an audience, listening to a variety of speakers and meeting new people.

After the conference, we returned back to the apartment.

As the days flew by, we all explored cafes, canals and little eateries, enjoying all Amsterdam had to offer. We arranged to meet some of the speakers from the conference, at one of our favourite cafes. We had in-depth conversations about metaphysics, law of attraction and energy while sipping tea and laughing at each other's jokes. We walked back to our apartment together, inviting them in to have yet another cup of tea.

The organiser of the conference leaned in towards me, "So what are your plans for your future Anja?"

I told him about the modelling contract, and how it was being finalised and I was planning to stay in Amsterdam, seeing where it would take me and what modelling work I could do.

"Where are you going to stay?" he asked me, knowing there were only four days until my flight was due to leave back to Australia, and I still had not cancelled my tickets.

"I don't know yet," I replied confidently, "I am sure I will be able to attract it as long as I don't worry about it."

Really, I had bigger things to worry about. I had not heard back from the agency yet to confirm the contract and that I should stay in Amsterdam. My flight was FOUR DAYS AWAY. I had not cancelled it and I had not arranged accommodation.

There was not much longer I could wait, I really needed an answer there and then.

Mum and Alex knew that I was stressing, so I emailed the agency asking them what was happening, and if I should stay there for the fashion season. I explained my situation – that I would be needing to cancel my flights and book accommodation as soon as possible.

Similarly, to what I did the first time at my modelling casting, I knew I had to get happy, relax, trust in myself and do my visualisation.

I visualised getting the contract, signing it and jumping up and down in excitement. Before I could finish the visualisation, I was blinking my eyes open into the morning light.

We were checking out of the apartment today and spending our last few days in Northern Holland with MFL.

We explored a few of the towns dotted along the way to their house – lush green trees, cobblestone footpaths, decadent churches and character homes – it seemed like they were villages from fairy tales.

Eventually, we arrived at his house, resembling a home from a Hans Christian Andersen novel. The weather was "warm", equivalent to that of an Australian winter which sprung all the flowers and trees into bloom. There was the smell of crisp European air – newly trimmed lawns and florals laced with freshly brewed coffee. His backyard led to the water – narrow canals weaving through the backyards of these European homes, as well as paddocks with sheep, horses and cows.

We dropped off our bags and picked up a picnic to have on his boat while we got changed. I knew it was about 18 degrees, but I have always wanted to be on a boat in a bikini, even with the now overcast, grey skies.

As we took off from his jetty it began to sprinkle down rain. We had some food on the boat and looked out at the backs of all of these beautiful houses and green fields with long lilac-tipped grass blowing in the wind. MFL's wife climbed out onto the edge of the boat into the weather grasping my phone tightly, as I shakily tried to balance as I tiptoed along behind her to get to the bow of the boat to take the perfect photo.

I stood as still as I could to get a few happy snaps, before returning into a jacket and towel back in the boat.

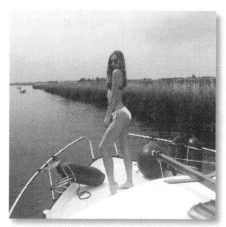

On the boat

After our sail through the canals, we went inside, and I connected again to WIFI, seeing messages from friends and emails popping up. I saw an email from the agency saying they were going to send my photos through to some clients and get some castings lined up and were happy for me to stay in the Netherlands for fashion season. I also saw another message through my model page on Facebook from the conference organiser inviting me to stay in his house in the Hague with his son, while he was abroad.

Without having to stress about accommodation, an offer fell in my lap.

I had never lived with anyone (apart from my parents) in my life, so was nervous about the offer but really grateful that it had come up. Now I could relax – my accommodation sorted, modelling contract sorted, and I was in a beautiful house with two of my favourite people in the world.

Seemingly without a worry in the world, mum and Alex waved goodbye to me with a smile, doing the royal wave behind them as they went through to the customs area at Schiphol airport.

Ok. Wow. I am in a country, all by myself.

MFL kindly drove me to the Hague – my new home for however long I would be there. I did not know *anything* about the Hague. Blame it on being a high school dropout, but I had no idea it was home to the International Court of Justice, the International Criminal Court, the councils, courts and cabinet of the Netherlands, foreign embassies or a major city to host the United Nations. There was a lot I did not know, but I had a lot of time to learn.

We arrived at the apartment block where I was going to be staying, and I buzzed on the number of the apartment and heard a kind male voice answer, inviting us to come in. I walked inside, greeted by two levels of stairs – four flights in total. I am not complaining about all the stairs; I am just complaining about my 35kg bag I had to drag up there. Lucky for me I had help with it, so I was only carrying an oversized handbag feeling like it was weighed down by a tonne of bricks.

I feel sorry for the son, having this strange 17-year-old girl from Australia with an older man hauling a huge suitcase up the stairs behind her, coming to take over his space. He stood at the top of the stairs, waving and smiling and gave me a welcoming hug hello on arrival, and I immediately thanked him for letting me stay. He was a good looking, blonde, 20-year-old Dutch boy and the thought of just meeting and then moving in together was daunting.

I shyly walked through the door, examining every inch of my new home. There were Tibetan colours decorating the lounge and dining room, with Buddhas, a prayer table and plants. I felt right at home in such a peaceful environment. I was staying in his father's room that had earthy red walls and big windows opening out to trees that lined the streets.

The bathroom was beautiful, with big black tiles. The toilet was in its own small room with a doorway entry from near the kitchen, and another leading into the main bathroom that had another access point off the son's room. I knew I would have to try and time my washouts for when he wasn't in the house, as the toilet was so close to both his bedroom and the kitchen, and I was shy.

My new housemate and I began chatting, sharing many laughs and making basic small talk. We decided to walk down and get some groceries together, and I insisted that as I was not paying any rent, that I pay all grocery costs for the both of us.

My sense of direction not being the best, I blindly followed my housemate as we walked through what seemed like a maze of streets, to the grocery store. I always get tricked into walking places that are "not far", but I can guarantee this short walk was at least 1-2 kms just to get there! AND THEN WE HAD TO CARRY THE GROCERIES BACK!!!

We both just bought our own things, we were going to cook something nice together but from memory we ended up giving up on that idea! Maybe it was a sixth sense on his part that I am not the ideal domestic goddess.

By the second day, my housemate had left the house to go to college. It was the perfect opportunity to go have a washout, so I dragged my big bottle of glycerol that MFL, who is conveniently a doctor, sourced for me, and dug up my catheter tubes and stole the salt from the kitchen. My wash out went well, and after an hour or so I was confident that I was 'clean' enough to leave the house.

The following day was my first casting in Amsterdam, so I thought it would be a good idea to go for a walk, get to know the neighbourhood area and get some exercise. I put on my active wear and was ready to go. There was just one problem.... I could not work out how to get out of the house.

Yes, there was a door, and no I wasn't being held captive.

I just could not work out how to open the door. It was some sort of strange Dutch door opening mechanism my Australian brain could not comprehend. It was probably designed in some incredibly efficient way that the Euros are known for, but I was used to overly complicated Aussie designs.

I tried everything... pulling, banging, twisting, pulling in different directions, pushing, shaking. I was stuck.

What does every 17-year-old do when they are stuck and need help.

"Mum, I am stuck." I typed out in a Facebook message to her all the way across the world from me.

Mum doesn't usually use Facebook, but I had encouraged her to use it to contact me while I am overseas. It was a win – win situation. I won in the sense that I could talk to mum easily, and also won in the sense that I had free entertainment watching what mum did on Facebook – join activism groups, post photos of the sky with the caption 'Chemtrails' and comment on her friend's new profile pictures "Wow, you are one smoking hot mama" as well as occasionally write me private messages and post them on my wall by accident. She really needed supervision.

Mum clearly leapt into action – trying to assess the situation as best as possible and work out if I was in danger.

"I can't get the door open to leave the house, do you have any ideas??" I typed to her, attaching a photo of the door.

She interrogated me on all the ways I had tried to open it, as I went by each one step by step, for the fifth time.

The little three white dots were moving, before a message popped up, "let me google Dutch lock mechanisms and we can try work it out"

She sent me a photo from Pinterest of the same lock (that had earned its place on my greatest enemies list over the past two hours) to which I replied, "cool photo, but now what?"

I was trying to tell mum my housemate could just teach me, and I would stay inside until he got back home and just do some indoor exercises, like my favourite - the 7-minute workout - or whatever else was trending online.

Mum replied, "Found a lock like it... Now let's see if we can find how it works... Don't want him (housemate) to see you as sh*t-for-brains" - thanks mum HAHA.

To cut this great tale short, SOMEHOW mum managed to research "how to open Dutch door lock" and sift through until she found the right answer. I was FREE!!! But by then I had lost the motivation to go on the walk, so just went back into my room to do some exercises myself.

I spent that night working out the Dutch transport system. I spoke to my housemate about it and I found the transport Journey Planner and set to work. My casting was at this huge fashion school in Amsterdam, and I had to plan how to get there from The Hague. I worked out the fastest way was to walk to the bus stop, take a bus to the train station, take a train then switch to a metro and then walk 600m or so. I did not have any data on my phone, or an international sim, so I had to just screenshot the directions and hope for the best. I realised that with no phone data, I wasn't even able to access maps on my phone, so I really had to study the directions and rely on myself.

I woke up that morning, showered, dressed in fitted jeans and a tight khaki top I had bought in a small town in Northern Holland and slicked a light layer of mascara onto my lashes. I had been practicing with the door handle, so was happy to be able to let myself out on time.

Checking my phone at every transport interchange, and double checking every detail, I made it safely to the place I was supposed to be, walked inside and gave the designers name for them to notify that I was there. It was a fitting for a big runway show for the designer's graduation and if I did well at this fitting, I would book the show.

The designer came up to collect me and led me downstairs to the fashion rooms and design studios. He explained the futuristic concept of his collection - a city that had survived an apocalypse and race of people that had emerged from the water, or something along those lines. I got out of the clothes I was wearing and was helped into this dress made of pure plastic, material resembling that used for a tent cover.

It was cold out but in the dress it was quite warm and I felt insulated by the material. There were little drawstring features and it was very futuristic. I was given a cork belt that resembled a horseshoe to give the dress some shape, and heavy flat men's shoes, painted a steely blue-grey colour and dusted with sand.

I saw some other models filing in, some that I recognised from my agency's website, so I introduced myself and waited until we were called in to the judging panel to assess the designer's outfits.

Finally, we were called into the room. One model behind the other, four or five of us walked in a line, all standing straight and equally distanced from each other.

We were standing very still in a line, letting the judges walk around us, feel the material of the clothes and examine the details of the design. We had to be frozen like in a game of musical statues, only to move when asked.

The judges went back to their panel and instructed us to stand forward one by one and turn around to show the details of the clothes once again. I was second from the left, meaning once the first girl went forward and returned, it was my turn.

I confidently walked forward, the shoes heavy and weighing my feet down. It was hard to walk elegantly in such big sandshoes.

As soon as I returned again, I was back to standing still. I really wasn't feeling too well. By this time, it was the early afternoon and to allow for the travel time to get there, I had left around 8am. I hadn't eaten, as I was so busy getting there and did not want to bloat as I was unsure if I would be measured again or if I would have to wear anything tight.

I was beginning to feel flushed with heat and unstable in my stance. I could not expect that this was because I hadn't eaten, as I had been through periods of not feeling the need to eat and it had never made me sick before.

A wave of exhaustion flooded my body, my skin was cold and clammy to touch but felt like it was burning internally. My heart was racing, and head felt like it was spinning. I tried to ignore it. I was scared for anything to happen to me and am only realising now that I did not have any travel or health insurance anymore, as we had cancelled my flight home and I had outstayed my cover period.

I was feeling dreadful but knew that my housemate couldn't pick me up as even if he wanted to, he didn't have a car. If I could somehow manage to contact MFL I could maybe get some help... but he was about 2 hours away from where I was, and if he were to take me home as well it is adding another 120km to his travel. I was on my own with this...

I just had to focus on staying up right, present in the moment and ask my guardian angels to help me. I was just feeling worse and worse. I did not want to say anything as I REALLY wanted this job, and I couldn't ask for a chair or leave as it wouldn't make me look like a reliable and professional model.

My head spins were increasing. I tried to sway my body to improve the blood circulation in an effort to improve my condition. The judges were still assessing the models down the line. I really tried to hold on as long as I could, hopefully only ten minutes or so more.

I couldn't. I started getting black blurry dots in front of my vision. I tried blinking them away, but they just clouded my sight more and more until it was pure black. Suddenly my hearing cut out completely along with my sight, one of the models beside me catching me on my fall to the ground.

My eyes opened again quite instantly, and I could see with blurred vision. My limbs were jelly; I could not support my body or stand up. The designer rushed and got me a chair, someone else got me water and the judges passed me two pills. "What are these?" I murmured, unsure of their treatment plan.

"They are sugar pills, to get your energy levels back up again," I was told "take them".

I swallowed these pills and sat for a minute or two, before insisting I was fine to stand up. I was so embarrassed. Thoughts were running around in my head – I was concerned I would get a bad reputation, wouldn't book the job or even worse, that my agency would drop me all together.

Once I was standing up again, the onset of these symptoms took over, landing me with no sight and hearing for a second time, as my body was guided back onto the seat. I stayed seated for the rest of the casting until it was complete and the models could leave the showroom.

"I am SO sorry," I apologised to the designer, "that has never happened to me before..."

He told me that it was okay, and these things happen to models all the time – it is almost expected.

All the girls from my agency at that casting and I were asked to go and meet our agent in the city in Amsterdam. We were running behind time as the casting had ended later than expected. I was glad to be with Amsterdam locals who knew their way around. We all got dressed back into our clothes and put our coats and scarves on and went out into the crisp air once again.

After navigating the city, we ended up in this beautiful high-end cafe/restaurant that had exposed brick interior, extravagant lights hanging from the ceiling, and a mezzanine floor where you could sit up and look out to the street through big historical windows. We sat down on big black leather chairs and lounges on this level and met our agent.

We discussed everyone's jobs and what was coming up. My agent emailed me through an official contract to complete and let me know that she had got confirmation I had been booked for the show that I just cast for. I was so happy with this outcome and felt so comfortable to be included in this agency meeting with such stunning models.

Afterwards, I had to navigate back to the nearest train station, as I thought once I got there I could find out what train goes to the Hague. One of the girls had to go to the train station too so we walked together, catching another tram, and making it to the central train station of Amsterdam.

The train station was so huge, and most of the platforms were divided into two sections, with a different train operating from each end. I had to be incredibly careful to ensure I got on the right train, as I was not used to this system at all.

I was so relieved to be home safely, after catching the bus from the train station and getting to the front door. I MADE IT. I blacked out twice, but now I am home.

I went to jam my key in the lock of the common door downstairs. It slid in perfectly but would not turn. I jiggled the key around, sliding it in a bit further and trying to move it, even pulling it out slightly and jiggling more. NOTHING WOULD MAKE IT TURN.

How embarrassing. I pressed the button to buzz up to the unit and there was no answer. Oh god.

I tried again with the lock and key, but nothing would work. I sat in a heap next to the door, waiting patiently for someone to arrive at the building, or for my housemate to come home so I could get in. I had nothing to do on my phone as the distance was too far to pick up the wifi. I just had to sit patiently.

Anyone who knows me, understands that patience is not my strongest virtue. After waiting about 20 minutes, I tried again with the key in the lock. Still no luck. I buzzed one of the people in unit 1, telling her that I was staying there and wasn't able to get through the front door as my key didn't work. She buzzed me in without asking questions.

I felt so accomplished.

That was until I got up to our unit door, and that would not open either. This time I could turn the key, but I definitely could not open the door. I tried both keys on the key ring, and neither would work. I tried pushing and twisting, jiggling the key, jiggling the door... everything I could think of. Yet again, this lock defeats me.

I give up. I knock on the neighbour's door and enlist their help to open the lock. Bingo, they did it with the same key I was using, on their first try. I thanked them and apologised for being so hopeless! We shared a laugh before both going into our own apartments.

I was home. Now I could relax.

XIX

—⚯—

Tenacity

Do not wait for opportunities to present themselves, create them

I began getting bookings in the Netherlands, as confirmed by a message from my agent.

I was happy to get booked for a shoot so soon and began mapping out how I was going to get there – bus, then train, then metro, then bus, then tram and then a 500m walk. It was daunting when I could not even access a live map on the way and travelling by public transport in an unknown area. I had to keep watching and listening out to the names of the stops, as I had no chance of seeing anything familiar that I could recognise as where I needed to get off.

I had a relaxed day at home with my housemate – chatting, laughing and getting to know each other. I just wanted to spend the day in warm pyjamas and relax to try and restore my body as I did not want another black out moment like the previous day. I was finding it hard to understand what could have gone wrong as I had never experienced a blackout like that ever before.

I admitted to my housemate my experience the previous day, and how I was unable to get through either of the two doors. He took me downstairs, and taught me how to get in. It turned out that both of the two keys I had been given could fit in the lock, but only one would turn. When I had got the first key in and it fit so well (even though it didn't turn), I assumed that it must have been the right key, as usually if it isn't, it won't go into the lock in the first place!

The apartment door was a bit trickier, you had to lift the door while turning the key, and then push - a complex combination for my simple-lock-trained brain.

The next morning, I confidently left the house, knowing that I would be able to get back in on my return.

Arriving, I walked into the big, white photographic studio, natural light flooding the space from the skylights above, sweeping high ceilings and makeup mirrors with a bench to one side. I introduced myself to the team of three, while one of the girl's salt-sprayed my hair, fluffing it up to give texture, and the other applied a light kiss of natural makeup on my cold skin.

They explained they had the idea of creating a #ReadyAF campaign – with AF representing the brand as well as "as f*ck". The first video was creating the cocktail "Sex on the Beach" wearing the brand's summer dress over bikinis.

I am admittedly impractical with anything involving the kitchen, so I knew my inner actor would really have to make an appearance here.

Once that was complete, a male model came in for the next video shoot. For this one it was about taking the perfect selfie and was to incorporate casual clothes as well as active wear. They decided that each instruction for taking a selfie, would translate to an exercise or yoga move. At the end they told me I would have to shake my bum up, trying to get the guys attention who is overly focused on taking a selfie of himself, while the camera goes out to the overall picture, of him and I side by side.

This male model looked like a Ken barbie doll and was interacting mainly in Dutch with everyone else, while I was getting changed into the active wear.

I would usually not be very flexible either, but I was hopeful that my long walks and a few stretches here and there could shine in this moment.

I discreetly bent over to touch my toes when no one was watching to see if I could touch them without bending my knees. I could make it. Thank god.

I went on set, moving from position to position fluidly, trying to execute it to the best of my athletic ability. I thought I did pretty well considering I hadn't done most of these moves for a few months now. Thank goodness for muscle memory!!

By the end of the shoot, I had a conversation with the male model as he sipped the 'Sex on the Beach' I just made, before saying my goodbyes to the team, thanking them for the day.

I set off again on my transport journey, making it home after two and a half hours! One of the rail lines to the Hague was out of use, meaning the trains were cancelled midway through the journey, and we were all diverted to buses.

There were so many people rushing to the buses, and we all packed in shoulder to shoulder. As the bus thinned out I was able to sit and ended up near a Dutch man who sparked up a conversation. He gave me his details on WhatsApp and offered that he could show me around a bit. I innocently thanked him for his kind offer.

When I got home, I noticed something in the foyer that I hadn't before. There was a Danish design cedar table, with an intricate design in the legs and sides that could fold down. Mum had the exact same table!! She had bought it at an antique auction in Brisbane, and it now had a place in our home. Now in the place I was living, this identical table appeared. I perceived this as a sign that I was on the right track.

When I came into the apartment, my housemate was there. I was telling him all about my day and he was sharing his with me too as we laughed together telling stories. We were having a celebratory night and as I could not have much privacy in the house, I was too embarrassed to go off into the bathroom, carrying my supplies and have a washout.

My bowels felt okay, so I didn't worry much about missing my washout, I just enjoyed my night.

In the morning, I was being picked up by my housemate's mother to go out as she had a day planned with me. I was so glad that I had someone else to spend time with and show me around.

I put on an appropriate, casual grey tee, khaki tight pants, boots and a jacket wanting to make a good and down-to-earth impression. His mother was gorgeous, tall, lean and with short, wavy blonde hair. We greeted each other with a smile and a hug and both felt immediately at home in each other's company. We went downstairs and got into her car and conversation was flowing.

We talked about everything you could image and loved being together. She took me to this beautiful animal farm outside the city centre of the Hague. There were beautiful small roads with blooming small yellow flowers, sweet country fences and cows in the fields.

We arrived at the farm, made for people to come and view the animals, with a souvenir and product store, restaurant, little boats in a small canal for rent and different barns with animals - big and small. All the animals were happy, comfortable and had huge spaces and opportunities to free-roam.

We went through each of the barns, wandering around as children played and live music filled the air. We stopped into the product store and bought two bottles of milk to feed the baby goats. These tiny little goats were running around in little groups, so soft, sweet and excitable. When you came near them, they would all run for you, wanting a sucker of milk. I was patting them as their sweet little heads twitched as they sucked and swallowed the milk.

We went back to her place, beautifully decorated with white and a few powder pink features. It was a place where I would love to live – European, light, white and homely.

We continued speaking, as we prepared a salad together in the kitchen, and brought it into the outside area to enjoy in the sun. As we ate, my stomach was still gurgling as I enjoyed the different flavours in the salad.

My housemates mum drove me home as my stomach gurgled along the way. We had been talking about my illness when dropping out of school and my experiences, so she understood that my health was not at its best. I was clutching my stomach as it made noises – feeling like I had food poisoning or that my bowels could give way at any time. I was holding in as much as I could, what felt like wind.

I was so scared it would end in disaster, as we were ten minutes away from home. I was praying to whoever I could think of - the universe really. "Please help me, help my stomach, make sure nothing happens, please" I was repeating in my head. Over and over.

With a maternal instinct, my housemates mum looked over at me, asking if I was okay. My palms were sweaty, and all the colour had drained from my face. I told her my stomach just did not feel good.

We were about T minus 7 away from the apartment. I was just focused on trying to keep my stomach. Suddenly, my stomach contracted painfully causing me to gasp and eyes to widen, as my tight jeans filled with warmth.

My nightmare finally happened. Sh*t in the car of the mother of a boy who I'm trying to impress. There was NOTHING I could do. It *really* happened.

She looked over at me concerned, "Are you okay??"

"I am so, *so* sorry," I paused as she looked confused "I just got diarrhoea in your car" I said to her.

I continued to apologise and blush in embarrassment on the way home as she assured me it was okay. I was still writhing in abdominal pain and feeling weak.

When we got to my place, she asked me if I needed a hand or anything. I politely declined and apologised again, slipping in "please don't tell your son."

I wrapped my jacket around my waist and proceeded to unlock the door and walk up 4 flights of stairs with it leaking down my legs. I just prayed that no one was home, so I could deal with this, shower and do the laundry in peace and privacy.

This prayer was answered, as I walked into the empty apartment. It's a shame my previous prayer didn't work though as that would have been a much better outcome.

I managed to clean myself up, and I was taking my clothes off when I got a call from my agent. Caught with my dirty laundry around my ankles I moderated my tone to seem chirpy and counteract the echo of the bathroom tiles. She told me a sister agency in Milano was interested in me, and I had to take new digitals as soon as possible, and gave me careful instructions on what they were looking for.

I told her I would have them to her first thing in the morning, and I cleaned myself up and was excited for what the future held. I got the digitals to her the following morning, after my talented housemate took some of the best ones yet.

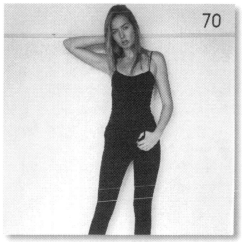

My new digitals

On my days off I explored the city in the Hague or went and explored new places with my housemates' mother.

In the city, I went from shop to shop, enjoying how beautiful it all looked – every building had character and charm, with each shop thoughtfully laid out. I felt at home in Denmark, and the similarities between the two cultures made me feel quite at home in the Netherlands too. There was some kind of familiarity there.

Going to the beach in The Hague I was blown away. Australia is a country with the best beaches in the world, but the Dutch were far ahead of us in maximising the enjoyment of it.

There were sunbaking chairs lining some areas of the beaches, clubs, bars and restaurants, with huge umbrellas and outdoor areas built on the sand. It looked like something out of a movie. We stopped by one of the restaurants and got an ice tea, as for one of the first times since being in Holland, I actually felt warm from the sun!

After that we picked up some photos and comp cards I had to get printed professionally last minute, with agency logos ahead of my castings the following day.

I was thrilled for my agent to let me know I had been approved for two fashion week castings. To get into a casting, the designer had to pre-approve different models to actually come along, so getting to a casting in the first place was confirmation you made it past the first cut.

Arriving at my managers before the casting to pick up my agency portfolio, I walked up to her apartment with a stunning model following behind me in the stairs. We both were measured again. They were telling her that her measurements were too big, and she really had to stick to a strict diet.

When I got measured, they wrote the measurements down on the page. I asked them, "Is there anything I need to change?". They said to be the ideal sizes, I would need to lose 1.5cm on my hips, and 2cm on my waist. I didn't realise that my sizes were slightly bigger than they wanted however got on with it as this goes with the profession.

I fitted out my new portfolio book and it looked great – I was so happy with how it was presented and loved my comp card.

I went together with the other model to the casting in one of the inner-city fashion houses. It was one of the designers for fashion week that would showcase on July 9th.

We met some of the other girls I had seen at the previous casting I went to, and we all cast one by one, in a white painted long room, with beautiful timber floors - walking up and down and handing across our comp card to the casting panel.

I walked confidently and felt happy with how the casting went. I had learnt that you really never know if you will get the job or not, until they tell you and put it in writing. For that reason, I could not make a judgement on whether I thought I had it or not.

I really enjoyed my time bonding with the other models and was feeling happy and welcomed.

The next day, I was back on a train to Amsterdam to another Fashion Week casting, that would also be held on the 9th of July. Because of the timing, I would only be able to book one of the shows.

The fashion house of the second designer, was a two to three level terrace house on one of the canals in the red-light district. I had found out that the girl from Germany had been accepted for the casting too, so I arranged to meet her and share a meal with her after.

I had to take a new train changeover, and eventually made it there after walking from the train station, trying to follow the maps to the best of my ability. I was there early, as usual, as I had left too much room for travel time.

I paced up and down after finding the right place, as I was there so early I waited to see other models turn up and walk in before I soon followed.

When I buzzed on the bell at the fashion house, the shoe designer answered, welcoming me with a warm, English accent. I introduced myself to him and the designer immediately, thanking them for inviting me, emphasising how excited I was to be there, and that I had come from Australia.

I saw some of the girls in front of me cast, as they were watched critically by the casting team. One of the girls came in with ripped jeans as it was such a raging trend. She was asked if she had fallen over, or how else she could explain the rips in her jeans. Obviously, the judges were not impressed with this clothing choice at all.

By the time it was my turn, I strapped on a pair of heels, ready to walk. This designer was very well known for incredible footwear with big and occasionally lethal high heels.

I was confident walking in heels, so I didn't worry much, however these were in a whole new ball park, thinner and taller than any I had seen before. They were more like a weapon. My walk was professional, and I was shining. I wanted to show my determination without having to open my mouth. When I turned back to the judging panel, the designer winked at me and I noticed the other judges were beaming. I was in with a chance.

I had such a good feeling about the casting, and was amazed by the place that I was in. There was a mezzanine floor in the terrace house, and everything was painted white, with a large white chandelier hanging in the centre of the space. There were sewing machines, beading stations and haute couture designs being worked on, lining the walls. It was such a surreal experience; one I could not have ever even dreamed of.

I waltzed out of the house, happy at the experience and playing in the thought of walking for that designer at fashion week. I waited for my German friend down the street a few metres away. I decided to indulge myself in some free wifi, the closest candidate being the local marijuana shop. I needed to contact the German girl, so I lurked around in the wifi zone outside sending her a message over Facebook.

As I was waiting, I was approached by a man, who chatted me up, asking me to go on a date with him. I felt uncomfortable, trying to be polite and friendly while remaining disinterested in his offer.

Before he had approached me, I saw him wandering up and down the alleys, eyes glistening as he examined the windows the red light district is most famous for. He didn't seem to receive my subtle signals so I tried being firmer.

Finally, I spotted my friend - the perfect escape. I excused myself from this man's company, running up to my friend, hugging her and wishing her luck heading into the casting.

I strolled up and down the street waiting for her to come out of the casting again. I saw the pimps looking me up and down, some of the girls in the windows looking threatened, and others smiling and winking at me. This was a whole new environment for me.

My next time in the Hague city centre, I was exploring a new area of high-end designer shops.

I wandered down the street into this sweet, family run and owned Italian café. I ordered a Chinotto as it reminded me of Sydney New Year's, where Alex and I discovered it in fridge at the house we were staying. I loved the flavour, and the memory, so ordered that and a homemade pesto pasta – my favourite memory from my childhood with my mum.

I sat in the bay window, looking out into the streets. I was approached by the waitress, we told each other our stories and got along really well. We exchanged phone numbers and agreed that I would come back there again and see her. She insisted that if I was ever in trouble just to give her a call.

I appreciated this notion of friendship and returned home with a huge smile on my face.

I had made friends with a few people through my travels, catching up with them on occasion when I had free time. I was enjoying all these blossoming friendships, however the Dutch boy I met on the bus and I were blown away, for him to learn I was only 17, and me to learn he was 35!!!!!

At home, I was eating ultra-healthy - having apple cider vinegar shots for my immune system and toning in the mornings, with my other meals being skipped or consisting of yogurt, sunflower seeds and dried white mulberries (superfood) or salads. If I am honest there was the occasional chocolate croissant as a celebration at the train station on the way home after not eating all day, or the delicious grilled cheese sandwiches my housemate would make for me on occasion.

As the jobs kept flowing, I was up early to head to the fashion school's huge production runway. Almost qualified as a professional public transport geographer of Holland, I found my way by multiple modes of transport once again.

I had been very nervous about the runway, as I was in the plastic dress again and was so concerned at the possibility of me fainting. Alex had been talking to me about kinesiology, and how plastic breaks the energy field of the body and weakens you. She explained to me doing a strength test, first normally, and then with plastic on my head I tested much weaker immediately.

I tried to figure out how to keep my body strong while wearing a plastic dress. Luckily, an idea sprung to mind!

I got all my little round crystals and shoved them inside my bra. I looked lumpy... voluptuous would be a nice way of putting it.

I believed it would make me stronger, so I just did it. It may seem crazy (it did at first to me), but I did not want to take any risks of blacking out and blowing it!

"Hopefully this will work!" I thought to myself as I grabbed my bag and head out the door.

XX

∞

Opportunity

The most important opinion should be the one you hold of yourself

I arrived, crystals in bra, to the huge performing arts centre where the runway was to be held. I saw many familiar faces with all of the girls in the agency I had got to know, were there with me.

The designer gave us all a pair of slides, and a funky cotton dress with a drawstring waist and our names written all over the material. It was such a cute idea and made us all easily recognisable to anyone else.

We were put into hair and makeup first. Hair was going to be teased up in a very futuristic way. They teased from the roots upwards. The hair that wasn't being ripped from my scalp was left looking frazzled - dead and unable to be resuscitated. One particular hairdresser had a flask in his pocket that he would take occasional sips from in between grabbing the models by the hair, jolting their neck back and ferociously teasing each strand. It was hard to stop your eyes from watering.

Unfortunately, in my case, the first tease done by the hair stylist just wasn't right, meaning that the head guy came in, ripping my hair out as it was brushed through violently, before re-teasing it to look identical to the first attempt.

The makeup was unbelievably light; a light coat of foundation and gelled eyebrows.

We went down to the rehearsal area. It was very structured, we would cue, and when it was our designer's turn, we would walk down into this huge open space before getting up on this moving platform, posed in a certain way. When it was our turn to come forward, we would be wheeled into the foreground, stopping before we each got off one by one, walking directly towards the audience before turning left to follow around the bottom of the stages perimeter.

We were then handed over to a runway coach, to watch each of our walks and ensure they all had the correct style to match the theme and each model walked in a uniform way. We first realigned our posture, worked on our style of walk, expression and routine. It was wonderful being with experienced models, and having a professional trainer ensure each walk was being executed to perfection.

The show kicked off with a bang, as we watched the other designers' model teams dressed in unusual outfits, knitted male G-strings and futuristic, 'Lady Gaga' themed fashion.

I was praised by my agent who came and watched the show, admitting that she was impressed. I raced home to watch the runway on the live video they had recorded.

A few days after that, I was notified that I had be chosen out of lots of models, to be one of the three to five girls chosen to cast for their brand. It was one of, if not *the* biggest online retailer in the Netherlands. They had a great reputation, and it would be steady, ongoing paid work.

I travelled 4 hours there and back in the rain for the casting, completely unfamiliar with the area. The office reminded me of a VOGUE headquarters, with the company's name in lettering on the wall. We headed down stairs to the photographic area where they took some test shots.

I felt confident in my body as I had been working out at home a lot as I wanted to keep in good shape, and hopefully make some progress towards my measurement goals. I was getting obsessed with the tape measure (I had gone out and bought one), it always being around my waist and hips at every moment I was at home, checking if I had grown or shrunk.

With the measuring tape showing no difference, I borrowed a yoga mat and took up bikram yoga. I found a funky studio, worked out the buses I needed to catch and where I had to walk.

It became my temporary routine. After fitting in a few kilometres walk, I would go to a 1.5 hour to 2-hour session of bikram yoga. I knew that this kind of thing could give me good results, as the previous time I had done it in Brisbane, I dropped a few kilograms just from one class, and I kept refuting that it was just lost sweat and water weight.

The session was difficult. I felt like blacking out numerous times and really just had to focus on keeping my body strong. My muscles would hurt as my hands and feet slid around the mat, struggling greatly to grip onto anything due to the sweat. I had to keep pushing my physical and mental boundaries and I would be sore and exhausted after class.

I was back there again the following day, determined to fit in even more long exercise sessions to get my body into some of the best shape it had ever been in. I did a morning class bright and early, as I was heading into Amsterdam later that day.

It so turned out that one of the girls I had met from my first ever runway in Brisbane, was in Amsterdam for a day as she was doing a tour of Europe. She had some free time so we arranged to meet. I was *so* glad to see a familiar face and share some Australian memories as we sat together, across the world from our homes.

We went to a restaurant in Amsterdam, and had a traditional Dutch meal, as neither of us had been enjoying the cultural food as much as we should have! It was delicious, a large meatball presented in a pool of gravy with mashed potato. What a dream.

We said a sad goodbye as she had to rush off and re-join the tour group.

In more exciting news, it was time for me to visit my agent again. After having an agency in India express interest in me, they had arranged a video conference for me to introduce myself.

I first said hello in my casting uniform of black singlet and dark jeans. As my agent discussed details, I slipped off to put on my black bikini before coming out, and letting them examine every inch of my body as I twisted and turned in front of the live camera.

The Indian agency gave me immediate positive feedback. They requested that I dye my hair brown as it would suit the Indian market better. I would do anything to further my career however would be sad to see the blonde go as I had now added the "blondes have more fun" mentality into my psyche.

I was sent through my Indian contract that evening. I was so excited I could not put into words. Once I got the contract however, my emotions transformed into nerves as I examined the strict terms of the contract.

I had to have a full body wax before arriving, have curfews and bedtimes each night, not be able to turn my phone off when I slept and have pay deducted if/when I was sick. I would have to share a room with many other girls, at least 4-6 models to one toilet. I could not really see how it would work with my health and washouts. Something about it just did not seem right. After mum lectured me about it being a "puppy farm", she decided that it would be best for my career.

As I was thinking about it, I was encouraged by both my mum and agency that it would be an amazing opportunity for me to build-up my book (portfolio), as there were a lot of fashion jobs available in India, that would give me the photos that they were wanting to see in Europe.

I was so happy that another agency wanted me, and the prospect of spending three months modelling in an exotic country was very exciting for me.

What wasn't exciting, was having my measurements taken again. I was joyous, telling my agent about all the hard work I was doing; back to back two hour workouts, walking and dieting.

I had gained two centimetres on my butt and waist. How could this possibly be? It is such a small amount when you account for the fact this 2cm could just be a big glass of water, but I was not at all happy.

My agent explained to me that doing any exercises on your butt, abs and legs wasn't good as it could bulk them up with muscle too much, and that would add size. I just could not believe I was working so hard, just to have that *annoying* measuring tape taunt me with increased size.

I asked her for suggestions on how I could lose that size, as I could barely grab a pinch of skin around my body as it was taut, tight and toned. She suggested to me both long walks and hula hooping.

Going home and researching, I was enlightened to the world of sports hula hooping. I went onto a reliable site and bought a very professional-looking hula hoop – one that weighed over 1.2kgs and had raised sections around the inside ring, so they would hit into you and stimulate the muscles and blood flow. I patiently waited for my hula hoop to be delivered while I deliberated with my mum if I should really take the contract in India.

I was able to get another opinion from a good friend who was a model in Australia that was on a Europe tour and in Amsterdam. I was so excited to have my second friend from home visiting my new 'home' in the Netherlands. We met in the city centre and indulged in fresh peppermint tea, with the stalks and leaves resting in the boiling hot water.

We discussed my opportunity with India and my experiences in the Netherlands. My kind Aussie friend and her sweet travelling companion shared their wisdom with me, giving me some good advice from a new perspective.

Saying another sad farewell to an Australian friend, she went off to re-join her tour as I got on the train back to the Hague.

Days flew by – more organic grocery shopping and salads, adventures into the city, visits with my new friend in the Italian restaurant and more.

I had a message from my agent wanting clear, no makeup selfies for the Indian agency. I had decided, despite the contract being very strict and some concerning things, I wanted to go for it. My main hesitation was that it was specified in the contract; if you left India even a day before the contract is complete (even from illness), or break too many of their tiny little rules, you would have your profit sheet striked to zero, and have to pay for all expenses without getting any of the income you had earnt. With my health, I knew that taking the contract would be a risk that I would be left with nothing but a bill after working hard and having to leave for health reasons.

I thought I just had to go for it and was encouraged by those around me to grab every opportunity with both hands. I had decided I would go to India, and the date had been set for July 15th - I would be going directly there from Europe.

I sent off the images back to my agent and unwrapped my new hula hoop. I was hula hooping over, and over, and over. I was determined to be the ideal size.

When I woke up the following morning I had bruises around my body from where the hula hoop had hit into me. I convinced myself I could see immediate results, and felt a sense of relief that I finally found something that would work.

I picked up the hula hoop for another round when I received a call from my agent. She was telling me that my contract with India may fall through as the agency there was concerned that my face was *too* fat.

Surprisingly, hearing this didn't affect me greatly, as at that stage my baby cheeks wrecking my opportunity was only a *possibility*. Whatever is meant to be will be. My face isn't REALLY too fat, *is it*?

I decided to relax and have a WO while my housemate was out, distracting myself from the possible fall-through of the contract.

Shortly after getting my mind off it, I received a second call saying that India had officially called off my contract, to travel abroad in just over a fortnight (I was in the process of booking in for vaccinations) as my face *was* 'too fat'. It was a kick in the guts, but that was just their opinion. I tried to stay relaxed and distract myself.

I got a third call, telling me that the fat on my face was becoming an issue preventing me to get more work. I was instructed to begin doing facial exercises and eating more foods that you have to chew more to exercise the chubbiness out of my cheeks. Maybe my face was fat because I wasn't eating much and not getting the exercise of chewing??

I knew I was getting this feedback from the goodness of their hearts to better me in my modelling career, but it was hard to hear.

This third call was the tip over the edge. Tears began running down my face. I was doing the absolute best I possibly could with my exercise, strict diet and very small meals *if any*. I had bruises all around my body from hula hooping too much to try reduce my waist and hip size.

I was googling diets and exercises for my face, doing them while sitting at the bench in the kitchen. I felt like these exercises weren't working. I felt *helpless,* like I had no power to change the appearance of my face at the request of others. I burst into tears - having my moment. My teary, snotty mess was interrupted by my housemate who arrived home and found me in the kitchen sobbing.

He was very concerned at what had upset me so much. I explained the whole story to him. He was livid and told me how polluted, wrong and toxic the modelling industry was. I could see the destructive side to it more now than ever before. You really had to be so strong in yourself to last.

There was a tiny part of me that was relieved I wasn't going to India. I had an off gut feeling about it from the beginning, otherwise I would not have hesitated at the opportunity. In my moment of upset I was judging the "fat face" thing as bad. In reality, it was the sign I had been asking for to direct me in what way to go - to India or home. I did not know the bigger picture of things.

Often we perceive things as bad when it doesn't go the way we wanted it to. We just have to understand that everything happens for a reason, and trust this reason is positive. If we treat things in an optimistic way, we heighten our vibration rather than wallowing in sadness that will just attract more experiences to generate the same emotion.

Of course, sitting at the kitchen bench crying, I couldn't quite see that.

XXI

<hr>

Playing in the big leagues

Never lose your belief in yourself

When I woke the following morning I had the perspective I needed. My tears were gone and I was highly focused on my goals. I understood that not believing in myself and my dreams as a model *now*, after another one of many rejections, would not make sense. I had no idea what was around the corner, what jobs I was being requested for at that moment and what was happening behind the scenes. I just needed to trust good things were coming and continue believing in myself (even thought it was hard at times).

If I had have given up after that, packed my bags and left back to Australia, I would have missed out on the next opportunity…

By 10am, I got the news.

I BOOKED THE JOB WITH THE HUGE ONLINE RETAIL STORE!!!!

AND, it would be REOCCURING work to shoot their website images. My face would be cropped out of the website pictures however it was a great job for me to book! I was so happy I was dancing around the house. I just had to confirm my dates for my planned trip home to Australia (I was very homesick).

In MORE good news, I was congratulated as I had been marked as an Option for the most extravagant show at Fashion week. I thought this meant I was a backup but found out that most are marked as options until they finalise who will be walking the runway. I was halfway there, but anxious as to whether or not it would be finalised as the show was quickly approaching.

I went to bed each night, doing my same visualisations. I visualised walking down the runway and getting the call to book the show. That was all I could possibly do. Visualise and relax that it will happen, without the expectation of it as the enjoyment of the possibility had already been experienced.

I was booked for another shooting in Amsterdam. I thought it was going to be a warm day, so I slipped into a short summer playsuit, wearing boots and bringing a jacket just in case. I arrived at the shoot, walking through another industrial looking area just near Amsterdam city.

I was in front of the camera again, completing all the remaining shots of the clothing when I got an urgent call from my agent through one of the photographers there. She had been unable to reach me as I did not have wifi and was uncontactable.

She told me congratulations, I had booked fashion week and now I just had to venture into Amsterdam city quickly, to go to the fitting.
!!

Without a moment for celebration, I bounced out of the studios ready to go to the fashion house. The photographers there had shown me a map on their phone of where the fashion house was located, and I had to take a photo and navigate the streets from Central station.

I hadn't taken the same route the last time I went there, so it was an unfamiliar walk. When I started to get into the red-light district, I noticed lots of men looking at me. My knee-high boots and tiny short playsuit that I was constantly pulling down was drawing the wrong kind of attention (yes mum, I should have listened to you).

I was in my nude underwear for the shoot, had basic light makeup and my heels with me just in case. If the call from my agent would have come in even half an hour later, I wouldn't have got it until well into the evening once I had returned home.

The timing was perfect, and I could not have been more excited.

Walking into the fashion house once again, as a model in the show I felt so tall, proud and grateful. I got on so well with the designer as well as the shoe designer. I went straight into the main room where I had my original casting, but this time it was alive, with people in every corner sewing on beads one by one, creating the most stunning haute couture designs.

I was put into outfit, after outfit, taking photos in each of them. Some of the other girls couldn't come to the fitting, so they were happy to fit the clothes on me as we were enjoying each other's company. They loved seeing how in awe I was of the designs. They had divided the show into good girl/ bad girl sections, and for the first time in my life, I was typecast as the bad girl. My look was a leather, crocodile body suit as a symbol of being from Australia (famous for Crocodile Dundee). I felt so special that they had put so much thought into what I was going to be wearing.

They could not stop giving me praise, as we got on with such great laughs. They told me that my body was amazing, as it fit all the clothes perfectly, filling them out how they were supposed to be worn proportionally and looking just right. They had taken my measurements at the original casting, so my outfit was already fitted appropriately to my body.

I saw the shoes I was going to be wearing, the only pair in the show with that particular design. They were long net boots up to my mid-thigh with a black ribbon seam in the centre at the front. This was sewn onto a high platform, with the heels only to balance on a thin, metal spike. I knew that the designer was famous for the crazy tall shoes. I had watched on YouTube a previous show from a few years before of three of the girls falling on the runway in these shoes, and someone had remixed it to music. This didn't do much for my confidence, but when I put on these boots, made for me, I couldn't have felt more self-assured.

They pinned the netting to the exact thickness and length of my legs. Everything was made perfectly for me. My hard work had paid off. *This was it.*

I left that fitting on the highest of highs. It was the 6th of July, the 9th was the show and the 10th was my 18th birthday.

Everyone I told was ecstatic at the news. I decided that I would head back to Australia after the show, and return to the Netherlands in mid-August/September for the online store work. I missed my parents, Alex, being able to drive, my dog Punky, my friends and everything I found familiar, even though I was beginning to get used to this new normal.

Everything was clicking into place. I had been speaking with my sister and for my 18th Birthday she was going to fly me over to Denmark to meet her and celebrate, as she was coming home from Croatia that same day. Mum then booked the flight for me home from Denmark. Again, it was so last minute, and was only done the night before the big runway, two days before I was due to fly.

We had put our apartment up for sale in Brisbane as we decided that we would like to be closer to nature and the trees, rather than the sirens, fighting, drunkenness and domestics of Fortitude Valley. My cousin was now heavily pregnant, and scheduled for a C-section on July 22nd, something I did not want to miss, *and* I had been invited to be on the judging panel at a casting for my agency.

Mum also sent me a message, asking me what I would like for my birthday. "Come on mum..." I wrote, "you don't need to get me a present after everything, and besides - if it is something from the antique auction I don't want it." She was addicted to the antique auction and I had no idea where else she would be looking for a present.

She sent me a link to a car. "Ha-ha mum very funny" I responded. We had spoken in depth previously about the possibility of me saving for a car and buying one for myself. She had been adamant that even if I would pay for it with my own money, we did not need two cars between us. I had given up on the whole concept, trusting it would all work out eventually.

Mum had found a car by chance online, stumbling upon it being auctioned in a few days' time. She only found it as she was trying to be nosey, addicted to Peugeots and seeing how much her Peugeot dealership jacked up the price in comparison to auction houses. She then saw my car and fell in love.

"This is your present" she announced. I couldn't believe it. I wrote back, "THANK YOU THANK YOU THANK YOU!!"

All my flights were booked and tomorrow as show day. In preparation, I had a double shot of apple cider vinegar, hula hooped for 40 minutes straight and wrapped my butt and thighs up in glad wrap with coconut oil thickly coated underneath.

Bright and early, I was up and out of bed, heading off to the Gashouder in Amsterdam where Mercedes Benz Fashion Week was held. I seemed to catch the wrong bus from the train station, getting completely lost and setting off on foot. I just looked at my screenshot map and started walking through these grass fields towards a more populated area, winding through parklands power walking so I wasn't late.

Finally, I found it. A sign pointing BACKSTAGE for fashion week. At the door my name was marked off, and I was given a MBFW lanyard with a card "MODEL" hanging off it. I knew this was about to be one of my most prized possessions as I was still in shock that I was there.

One of the other girls from my agency had been booked for the show, and another for a different designer that was showcasing an hour before we were.

We put our bags into the tent for our designer in the huge backstage area filled with bright lights and busy, rushing people. We found where each of our outfits and shoes were laid out, along with a photo of how they should be worn. I was in three of the photos from the fittings but was happy to see my name pinned to the black crocodile bodysuit and thigh-high boots.

We were pushed through hair and makeup. Makeup first – the style was dramatic, 1970s baby doll eye makeup, with the crease of the eye drawn in charcoal smudged eyeliner. As I had someone doing my makeup, I had one person painting my fingernails, and another painting my toenails a light grey-nude colour.

I was then led over to the hair area. It was at least 100 square metres just dedicated to the hair stylists. Our hair was all brushed over to one side, and thin layer by thin layer, it was pasted with gel flat on our heads, in a circular motion across the back of the head, centring in the crown.

I was intrigued with this look, interested to see what would happen. Once all the hair was glued flat, I looked like I had a blonde scalp on a bald head. They then put a nude bald cap over the top of our hair and told us just before the show we would get a wig put on.

I had a chance to try on the amazing shoes – now sewn up and made for my leg. I was a bit nervous about how they would sit, as I had developed red, raw blisters from my long walk through the field to get there and didn't want it to be rubbed on by the new shoe. I put a Band-Aid on as a precaution and slipped on my shoes.

They made me so extremely tall and threw off my balance a bit as I suddenly became 10-15cm taller and was trying to find a good equilibrium. The thin nail heel had no grip on the bottom, and we were trying to walk around on soft carpet. There were a few wobbles when walking on the uneven surface. How it would feel to walk on the slippery polished concrete runway was unknown. All that was certain was we would have to rely on our professionalism, training and balance for when we stepped onto the runway in the heels at showtime.

The problem with my shoes, was that when I walked the boot would twist around with my legs, meaning the black line up the centre would be far from straight. The shoe designer watched while I practiced my walk on the carpet, deciding that he would come up with a solution soon.

We all went out to see the space and rehearse where the show would take place. All the models sat in the front two rows at the beginning of the catwalk, while the runway director and designer explained the show concept... all in Dutch. Or most of it in Dutch anyway. I tried to tune in with my limited Danish ear and find some similar words, but I was at a loss, reading off body language and hoping there was someone in front of me I could copy off.

We went one by one along the runway, in the correct order and timing as a full rehearsal. In the centre of the runway there was this man hole, with a big, round concrete lid with a small gap between the lid and the floor, as well as a metal corrugated feature in the middle. In my normal shoes it was no big deal, but in shoes as tall and thin as what we were wearing, it was a screaming hazard for neck and back breaks.

On return back to the main area, we were hurried in to get our wigs on. These wigs were curled and styled in a typical 1960s bun and were a mixed shade of snow white with a touch of a fairy floss pale pink colour. The hair stylists glued the netting onto our scalp, ensuring the wigs were very well attached. We then had a mixture of netting, pink ribbon and fabric flowers hooked under our chin and tied up on the top of the hair. With identical hair and makeup, every model looked so similar.

The last hour in the tent was crazy; outfits having additional changes, repairs and finishing touches sewn, all the models were being dressed, sewn up and shuffled into the room behind the stage.

The solution for my shoes slipping down was solved, as ribbons were being sewn around my waist like a garter, with two ribbons hanging down that would be sewn on to the top of the shoes. They slipped on the leather jumpsuit very carefully over my head and hair, clipping it up between my legs. They checked with the designer, and as the leather was cold it had become shorter on my body, meaning it was slightly higher cut than what he wanted.

The designer spoke to someone, who quickly ran off, handing me some black hand sewn underwear to put under so if it came up more when I was walking, it would be disguised by the black underwear instead. I slipped those on as they sewed me into my shoes via the garter they had created. I knew then that it was go time, nothing could stop it from happening now. I was in my shoes, lining up and getting my wig sprayed and tousled, and face powdered.

I was standing in line, heart racing, with dressers between my legs pulling down the jumpsuit at my crotch to stretch the leather.

It was go time. The hand pushing at my back to indicate it was time for me to walk out. I already had my shoes strapped on tightly, and could feel that on the hard, cold, polished concrete floors I had no grip. At all. If you didn't hit the ground straight on the top of the nail, then you were about to go belly up.

I stepped out onto the catwalk, music playing with soft voices talking in the audience, as well as in the background of the song. As I walked, striding one foot in front of the other, shoulders back and head up I got goosebumps all over my body. I was exactly where I wanted to be. All I could see were the blinding white lights, causing the runway in front of me to look like a bright walkway, hovering in darkness.

Click. Click. Click. The sound of my nail heels tinkling the concrete before lifting up for another fierce stride.

I was relaxing into it, heart still pumping fast with adrenaline.

Pop Ohhhh crap.

Great models come from training. In that training we learn many skills and rules. We are taught that if we have a wardrobe malfunction, we need to just stay calm, continue the walk and by no means flinch, stop, fix it or leave the catwalk. My training was about to be needed.

The clasp holding my bodysuit together that they had been pulling on seconds before I stepped out onto the catwalk, popped open.

I could feel the elasticity of the leather spring it back to resting position, hovering above my crotch area.

The worst part was, I was one third up the runway, heading towards this obstacle grate in tiny thin steel heels and *now* my bits were hanging out!

I completed had forgotten I was wearing black underwear underneath and was so concerned that my nude G-string would have moved and was revealing something. Not quite how I thought I would be making my international fashion week debut.

I could hear chatter, unable to differentiate if it was the backing of the music, or the people in the crowd mocking. Every instinct in me was wanting to dash off the runway, cover myself or try and fix it up.

Instead, I didn't even flinch. Really it was a great distraction to ensure I glided over the floor effortlessly.

My mind contemplated whether I would be wanted to continue if my bits were popping out the bottom. I decided I just had to stick with it, so I did.

In a heartbeat it was over. I was backstage again with tingles, adrenaline at an all-time high. I was telling the dresser that my suit popped open, and he clipped it up again, and tested the pressure it could take, telling me it was all ready for the finale.

At the close of the runway, all the models walked in a cluster formation along the catwalk. I was in the centre in the middle of the pack, and just loving it. I had achieved what I had been wishing for longer than we could both ever realise.

Halfway along the catwalk, my jumpsuit popped open once again. What else could I do than continue to walk with pride?

I got backstage, concerned that I had let my agent down, and that I did not do well because everyone was too focused on the jumpsuit popping open. My housemate and his mum were there watching me, and they messaged to say they loved it. I messaged my agent, telling her what happened. They all told me, not only did they not see it pop open, they didn't even notice it.

Even now, words cannot describe how I felt in this moment. I learnt that all runways are similar, different places, faces, designs but the same feeling as you walk out of stage. My goal had been achieved. Now I could die a happy woman.

I went backstage, having my bodysuit sewn together, with one woman holding me upright and two sewing in between my legs. It needed to look good for the final group photos.

Once it was all over, I went to get my wig removed. I was planning on going to the Afterparty, but my hair was all glued to my scalp. One of the lovely hair artists tried to make it into a bun on the side of my head, but apart from that, not much could be done unfortunately. I blended in the black crease line on my eyelid, put on a white wrap around top and tight black skirt with some thin black stilettos. The strap of the stiletto going over the toes and the ankles was so thin that I knew after a lot of standing, it would begin to dig in.

That didn't matter, because right now I felt like I was floating. I went out, said hello and gave big hugs to my housemate and his mum. I invited them into the fashion week afterparty with me, as I had to say goodbye to everyone at least. They told me they were tired and were wanting to drive back home again now.

I wanted to go with them but also wanted to ride this event and feeling out. This moment had been building for such a long time I did not want to cut it even a single minute short. I went into the afterparty alone, looking for a familiar face. I was just going to say hello but ended up getting engrossed in conversation with the great shoe designer and his inner circle. I was getting to know this group of people and having a few laughs.

Someone from the crew offered to buy me a drink, and I told him that I wasn't 18 yet... there were just a few hours left until my birthday. He told me it was already dark, so it was fine.

I sipped a gin and tonic in my mother and Alex's honour, celebrating this time I had in Amsterdam. Music and laughing created a high-energy atmosphere and I was surrounded by a group of new friends.

Within half an hour, I had been brought into the VIP tent with my designers and other members of the fashion community. I was having a great time, laughing, networking and making friends. I was invited to sail on a boat with a group of them the following day but told them that I had to go to Denmark, then back to Australia the following day. They begged me to stay in Europe and have fun with them, telling me Australia was just a big island so far away.

I had such a great time however was reminded of how late it was getting as my feet had become swollen and felt like they were being mutilated by the heels I had on. I had a lot to do before I left the following afternoon. It was ticking close to midnight when I said my farewells to all my new friends.

The designer and shoe designer took me aside, telling me sincerely that it was a pleasure to work with me as I had been so grateful, dedicated and determined the whole time, and this had shined for them. They assured me that they thought I would have a successful career ahead of me. I was given some information about some agencies in London where they had contacts and encouraged me to sign with them. I took the cards gratefully, so excited by the prospect. Maybe even naively, I did not want to be disloyal to my mother agency that had taken me this far and kept those business cards safely in a memory box.

I understood everything was only my own creation anyway, but I wanted to sit back and see all I had created thus far, and just appreciate it.

I said my heartfelt goodbyes and wandered out to the street. I walked along the rickety pavement in the dark, with only my stilettoes to wear, as I had asked my housemate to take home my modelling bag for me, so I wasn't carrying it around the afterparty.

I went towards to light down to a bus stop, trying to navigate what one to take as I was definitely not walking back the way I came in – through a dark parkland alone.

Eventually, I arrived at Central station, and *just* managed to get the last train to the Hague that night due to arrive there just before 2am.

I collapsed into my seat. I was exhausted and my feet in agony. I was in a train carriage all alone. The train seemed to be abandoned and sent shivers down my spine. I undid my shoes, giving my feet some freedom as I could not deal with the discomfort a second longer. Connecting to the train wifi, messages began popping in from my loved ones at home.

By this time, it had ticked over to the early hours of the morning. The first few minutes of my 18th birthday. Mum sent me a happy birthday, congratulations and love. I was just so overwhelmed, to be alone and cold in the dark of a different country at night on my birthday. The stress of the past few weeks was releasing as I concerned myself with the thought of having to pack up my life from the past few months in a rush.

Mum had found the runway live streamed somewhere and told me she couldn't be more proud - I did so well. I thought she was giving me sympathy, consoling me about my wardrobe malfunction and told her the day's events.

I told her that I didn't want to be alone anymore, and wasn't enjoying being in a foreign, unfamiliar country solo for so long. I was longing for home, touch and familiarity. I crave companionship.

My eyelids were heavy and I was desperately wanting to collapse into bed, but I knew there was still another leg of my journey home. Once I got home it would take at least an hour to wash and brush out all the rock-hard hair gel.

I arrived at the Hague train station. I looked around the huge station, and there was no one but me there. It seemed abandoned too.

I heard some footsteps rushing behind me, a group of people had got off another carriage as I walked past. Before I knew it, I was surrounded by three dark-skinned men. They were asking me what I was doing alone? Where I was going? If I would like to come home with them?

I was terrified. I realised I didn't even know the number for emergency services or police, *even* if I was able to call them. I knew I had to put on a persona then, like I did when I stepped on the runway.

I told them I was going home to my husband who was a policeman and was waiting up for me. Cliché, but it was the best I could come up with. They snapped back that my husband never had to know about me going home with them.

They were lurking around me and trying to harass me further. "F*ck off!' I said to them firmly and confidently. I wanted to seem strong. I felt very uncomfortable and was trying to make clear that I did not want them near me. They just seemed amused and very persistent.

Mum always advised me to be strong and direct in these situations.

"F*ck off! I am not going home with you!" I screamed to these men.

XXII

---⁂---

Coming home

Life never happens to you, it can only happen through you

Eventually, the men got the message and left me alone. Checking over my shoulder to make sure they weren't still following me, I shakily walked up the stairs in my tight skirt and heels up to the bus stop.

Crap. It was around 2am. No buses ran at this time. I juggled around my things to find where I had put a little piece of paper with my address scribbled on it, before looking for a cab rank. I walked around, unfortunately in a similar direction to the group of men from before. I saw a line of cabs, and got into the one waving me over, feeling relief that I was safe.

"Wow you are looking very sexy tonight, where have you been?" this taxi driver said to me. WHAT IS GOING ON TONIGHT!! I really felt uncomfortable here too. I kept strong, and my policeman boyfriend story, saying I was 24 years old rather than a *very* fresh 18.

I got him to drop me down the street from my house, waiting for him to drive off before I walked as I was concerned he may follow me. I wasn't a scaredy cat, but I just was feeling very creepy vibes.

I dragged my tired legs in crippling heels, up the four flights of stairs to the apartment, bursting through the door and collapsing in the lounge. My housemate was still up, wanting to see me and spend time with me before I left. It was really sweet, as he came to me with the realisation that he would really miss having me around. We had a good run between us, many ups and downs shared. It was going to be strange not seeing each other every day, as we had been living together for a while now and had become used to it.

I got into the shower, washing my hair thoroughly, over and over with shampoo, and brushing it out with conditioner.

By the time I got into bed, it was 3:30am. I was exhausted, but just wanted to spend the time talking together with my housemate and reflecting on the time we had spent together. He told me happy birthday and that he and his mum had planned something nice for me in the morning, and we were being picked up at 8am. I was so grateful they had thought of me!

I hadn't even packed and was getting anxious as I had to be at the airport by 5pm, it was at least 30-45 minutes away and there was not a single thing organised with my luggage AND I was going out in the morning!!!!

I was given thoughtful gifts from my housemate and his mother when I woke before being taken out for an adventure. We got a tea in the morning sun on the city centre, before walking about a kilometre to a river cruise tour of the Hague. I was wearing yet another inappropriate pair of heels, as it was my birthday so why the hell not!

As we walked along, I realised my long navy dress was see-through in the light as it clung tightly to my figure.

I stepped down onto this small flat boat that went around the canals giving tours. As I sat down, my stomach began gurgling. This was the scary gurgle I recognised from the 'car incident'.

I was in a boat – no toilet, no escape, no option to preserve my wardrobe, or cover anything up, and no clothing protection (it was a tight & see-through dress) to hold anything in. I was becoming stressed as we floated around the canal, seeing the buildings, parklands and historical places. Every time we had to go under a bridge, we had to duck as the bridges were within a metre of the water surface.

My stomach was getting worse, I was doing my prayers, clutching my stomach and doing some reiki on myself to try and stop my bowels.

By the time we pulled back up to the jetty, it had been one to two hours with this stress of my bowels. It was a miracle I had made it through. I was glad to be on solid land again in running distance to bathrooms... hopefully. I learnt in Holland that they don't have public toilets!! You had to go into McDonalds to use the toilet, thinking you were so clever, but unless you bought something there, you had to pay a fee just to use the bathroom. This was not ideal with someone who shared my birth condition, but I had managed to keep it together for the time I was there (apart from the car incident).

We had an iced tea and looked over the canals before we ventured back to the car and drove home. I was glad to be back in the apartment and go to the bathroom. I changed into something more comfortable – jeans and a long-sleeved shirt and coat.

I had only one and a half hours, to pack up the last two months of my life in a suitcase. I left some things for my housemate; crystals, soaps, skin and body products. There was a lot that I couldn't take home, even a bottle of tanning cream. Trying to avoid it going to waste, I attempted to convince a 20-year-old male that he should test it out. I left a little stash of my clothes there as 1 - I was coming back soon, and 2- don't tell mum, but I couldn't fit it in my suitcase.

I detached the parts of the hula hoop, putting into my suitcase along with (most of) the rest of my things. I really just squashed things into my bag and sat on it with my housemate to zip it closed so I wouldn't quite call it "packing".

I waved goodbye to my old home, not knowing when or if I would be back.

We jumped on the train, and my housemate rested his head on my shoulder and fell asleep - he was not used to such early mornings...

When we got to the airport and I had checked in, we got pizza together and said a big goodbye. Someone took a picture of us hugging farewell before I waved goodbye and walked through the gates to customs.

I stopped into a duty free alcohol shop, wanting to buy my first bottle of alcohol ever – by myself as a gift to my sister.

I walked into the store, already lost and not knowing where to go or what to get. I barely knew a thing about alcohol. I thought I should aim for something traditionally Dutch, so I asked the store worker what he would recommend as a Dutch alcohol. He told me yes, saying "get Bols" which sounded a lot like balls with a Dutch accent. He walked me into this small back room, picking down two ceramic bottles with BOLs written on the front, for him to say, "1 Bols or 2?" - this was going to be the laughing story I would share as we tried this alcohol in Copenhagen the following night.

He told me it was like a schnapps from the Netherlands, so I hoped my sister and her husband would like it. I wasn't even IDed when I bought the alcohol, so was a bit disappointed not to show off that it was my 18th birthday.

As I was nearing the flight gate, and boarding had begun, my stomach started gurgling horribly, and I had to run to the toilet and only just made it on time. It was like I had food poisoning, and I was unsure if I would be able to fly in this condition. My whole body was red and hot, I had a racing heart, nausea, the black spots in my vision and this runny tummy. I just wanted to be home, so I said a little prayer (I'm not religious by the way!!), did my home reiki job and set on my way. Denmark here I come.

I was waiting at the Copenhagen International airport for a while as my sisters flight from Croatia was delayed. With minutes left of my birthday, my sister arrived and we jumped on a crowded train with all our luggage, as she presented me a birthday present, a stunning, rose gold Emporio Armani ring. I loved my gift and couldn't have been happier and relieved to be with my family.

I was able to spend a few great days in Denmark with my sister and her family once again, venturing into Copenhagen, exploring all the fruit trees and berry bushes in her garden, and driving over the bridge to Sweden for lunch and CINNAMON BUN (favourite thing) FLAVOURED ice cream.

Coming home to Australia was wonderful. I was so happy to see my parents, my friends, Alex, my new car, and just be in the comfort of home. I drove my new car with so much pride to visit all my friends. It was good to be home.

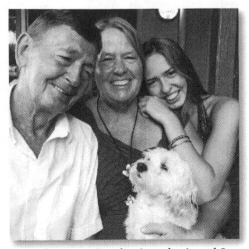

Dad, Mum, Punky (my dog) and I

I found a photo from fashion week of the designer and two models, and as you zoomed into the background you can see the people sewing up my bodysuit, with their heads between my legs. It brought me great enjoyment, giving my mum and friends a funny insight into the reality of life backstage of a fashion show.

Two days after arriving back home, I was in the swing of things, doing my hula hooping again and being a judge at a casting for my agency to recruit some fresh faces. It was a great feeling being there as a mentor and meeting all this new talent. I was able to share a bit about my modelling journey and give an insight into the agency and modelling as a profession. I was the agency's most successful model, having got an overseas contract and really followed my dreams within a year of starting. I was in a huge love bubble of appreciation for them and loved having another opportunity to work in the fashion industry as a mentor and trainer.

That night, Jasmine was taking me "out" for the first time. It was a rooftop bar with colourful lights on the ceilings, lots of attractive people, DJ and alcohol. I barely had anything to drink, only two or three over about 4 or five hours, so I was at a very mellow level. I didn't really see the point of excessive drinking for enjoyment. I wasn't wild, just sensibly observing this new environment before getting involved.

I saw many friends, and friends of friends that were asking me about Amsterdam, congratulating me and telling me how well I was doing. It was such an amazing feeling to have all these people that I wasn't incredibly close with extend an arm of friendship and engage in conversation when we bumped into each other.

I had a busy social schedule, seeing many friends, new and old, as well as great friends I had made in fashion. I was working on a project with John the photographer, playing around with ideas to start our own creative agency that can provide packages to clients. I needed to start monetizing my work more, as even though I was enjoying modelling as a career, having an unstable income impacted on my feeling of security and contribution to the household. I had to step up my game and get a continuous income stream.

On the 22nd of July, I had an amazing day with one of my best friends that I have known since I was three. We hadn't seen each other in a while and had recently reconnected. We had a beautiful day, exploring Montville, my old home town on the hinterland, having delicious meals and taking him for a wine tasting at an award-winning vineyard. Even though I could not have imagined having a better day, there was something more special about this day than an enjoyable time out.

It was the birth of my cousin's new baby. We had been around the family a lot during the pregnancy and felt very close to them and this new baby, so as soon as I got back to Brisbane, I went into the hospital to see them.

She was the most perfect baby I had ever seen. She had cute, delicate features, thick red hair, pale skin and had a sweet nature. When she was being changed by the midwife she was screaming, and as soon as I picked her up afterwards she was immediately comforted and fell asleep in my arms. We had a special bond that I could not describe, it was just such a beautiful feeling seeing new life come into the world, and especially a soul so innocent and loveable.

I was having a love affair with this baby, visiting constantly - at every and any possibility. I held her in my arms often, and we felt so happy and calm in each other's energy.

I was developing a mentor and trainer role within the agency and held two training days for both runway and photographic posing within a week, both with a good turnout.

I worked again on a few great projects with photographers that had become great friends in an effort to get more fashion work in my portfolio rather than commercial.

I had been home only a fortnight and had already done a lot with my modelling career. I walked for a fashion show for one of the universities in Queensland in front of the Editor of a top fashion magazine – a very exciting moment as being in this magazine has always been a huge dream of mine. At this event I played a large role in demonstrating the routine to the rest of the models. Most of them had been in the industry longer than I had and knew what they were doing, so it was a privilege to guide them.

One of the models from Australia that I had caught up with when we were in Amsterdam was walking at the runway too. I was glad to see her again and have a debrief on our trips.

The runway went off without a hitch, moving through look to look with ease, and having a good time as the rest of the models were from my agency so we knew each other very well.

Things were going well, I was busy shooting, booking runways, communicating with my agency in the Netherlands, eating well, discovering acai bowls and seeing my friends.

I was spending more and more time with my cousins little baby, and I was so honoured to be asked to be her Godmother. I loved this little baby before she was even born and had developed such a magnetic connection with her. I could not think of anything more special to me than her being my Goddaughter.

Mum was proud that this was a maternal role I could explore. Really, I had been trying to convince her that I wanted to find a boy and have a baby young, as I was incredibly obsessed with babies and pregnancy. I definitely had not found the right sperm donor, or ability to conceive since I was physically unable to have sex.

I had given up on boys as they created so much trouble. From the outside I may have seemed flirtatious, but behind closed doors I wasn't even doing my dilatations because I found teenage boys so infuriating and dilatations so uncomfortable. As much as mum said, "Oh just have fun with it!" I decided that both men and dilatations where things that needed to be navigated with great caution.

Since getting back from overseas, as soon as I slowed down, I began to crash. I had been so focused on modelling that as soon as my body had a chance to stop, I started getting sick again. This was likely to be due to being so run down. It is hard to believe that someone who "works" 3-5 times a week could get run down - but throw in exercise, planning for shoots and my poor record with health, it was the reality.

I was still having chronic abdominal pain, so I thought it would be worthwhile discussing with the doctors. I went for a CT scan and they could not see anything abnormal that could be responsible for my pain. I knew I wasn't making it up in my head, I just started to understand that sometimes doctors just don't know what to check, or what diagnosis to come to.

Throw in a few more fashion events, and I was off on a trip to Melbourne. The point of my trip was really to go with Jasmine to Melbourne for her to meet with a good modelling agency. We had planned our trip and were just holding off on booking flights and accommodation but had already set firm dates. I was wanting to go mainly for time with my bestie and to give her moral support. I let Mary, my agent, know that I would be down in Melbourne on those specific dates, and she booked me work - a bridal photography workshop and a magazine shoot with a well-known Australian label. I was incredibly excited about the opportunity, however was disappointed to hear Jasmine could no longer come on the trip.

It was too late for me to cancel now, so I packed my bags and set off. Mum and I were rushing from the apartment to the airport, and I had to drop my new car down into the parking space at mum's office as it could not be parked on the street due to parking restrictions.

Mums car park is a "3+ point-minimum turn in complete reverse" kind of park – one that getting into in a rush was almost impossible. Even though this was the millionth plane I had got on alone this year, I was getting a bit jittery about travel as I was worried I would miss the flight as I was running late. I decided to tackle the carpark from the back, and drive through it. It was a difficult space as there was a concrete ledge and metal pole on one side, and on the other side there was a huge concrete pillar.

I drove into the park on an angle, trying to think small thoughts to squeeze in (same technique I use when getting into small dresses). I cleared the front of my car around the pole on the far side, and thought to myself, "If the front is clear, the back is clear"

To be fair, I got this approach from my dilatations. If the front of the dilator could be pushed through the opening, that means the rest would fit as it is the same thickness. I didn't realise this doesn't work the same for cars.

I t-boned my car on this pole, scraping all along the side and landing a dint "across three panels" according to the smash repair place. I teared up and ran and told mum – we were both in shock and I was now miserable to have ruined my car already. At least it was parked though (finding the positive)?

Checking my watch, I grabbed my things and dashed off. There was no time to spare, I had a plane to catch.

XXIII

✦

Expansion

Always stay true to yourself, no matter what

The first day in Melbourne was the bridal shoot, and the other model, makeup and hair artists came to the Airbnb I was staying to get us made up. From there we travelled to a historical looking building and got changed in one of the hotel rooms there. Looking like a porcelain Russian doll with immaculate hair and makeup, I was dressed in bridal gowns with delicate white headpieces. The first dress I wore was see-through, with a while pattern on, and fell nicely around the shape of my body. There was then a netting skirt attached across each hip and my bottom, leaving the front with a simple silhouette of the original dress.

The other model and I got along really well – laughing, sharing stories and enjoying the time we were spending together. It was wonderful to meet such a down-to-earth model.

The following day was the big-time Australian designer magazine shoot, with the hair and makeup artists, and the second model coming to my house again. The hair and makeup was very 'fashion' with an Avant-garde feel to it. I knew this editorial was going to be amazing.

We went to this huge industrial area where a haute couture designer had a showroom, and we were going to be shooting in there. There were old fashioned leather sofas, stunning décor and magnificent dresses lining the walls.

We got out the big dress bag that was freshly picked up from the store and unwrapped it to see the designer garments hanging, ready for us to wear. The shoot went quickly and felt surreal as the location, team and clothing were spectacular.

After a big day shooting, and some excellent results, I was dropped back to the Airbnb. I was exhausted but managed to walk out to the shops and pick up a few small snacks, taking them with me to bed.

I was in Melbourne for another one-and-a-half days and was planning to enjoy my trip, catch up with some friends and also call into an agency in Melbourne to check it out. The Melbourne fashion industry is bigger than in Brisbane, so I thought it would be an opportunity to get some more paid work.

When I arrived at the agency, I was confident, presented well and got along with the agency Director. They took my measurements, and unfortunately my hips had increased by 3cm since I was in the Netherlands. Look at a ruler - it is nothing and distribute that around my body and its barely even noticeable. I had been working so hard and was trying to not beat myself up.

They told me my height and measurements, apart from my hips, were great, but unfortunately my hips were "too big for fashion", and I would get more bookings as a commercial model. They were wanting to sign me as a commercial model only, but I desperately wanted fashion. They told me they could of course put me forward for fashion jobs, however were unsure if I would be booked.

I let them touch my body, to feel if there was any fat I could lose on my hips and try and get into an exercise program. They felt around, only to tell me that "there is (was) no fat I could lose on the area, it is just the way you are built".

This felt like a kick in the guts. No matter how hard I worked, I could not get my hip size to decrease again.

Apart from a great trip to Melbourne, it had me thinking that maybe my size 6 body was just too big for fashion. I was torn now between pursuing modelling and going on a ridiculous diet and exercise program trying to change the size of my hips (even though I had been told by an agent it was impossible) or focus more on my health. I had a lot to think about it - was modelling still my passion? Was the industry still a place I wanted to be?

I realised the sexualisation, manipulation and destructive ideals that could rear their heads in the industry, as there are in most industries these days, and at 18 had to determine where I wanted to fit in. I wanted to be in a position where I could still stay true to myself while generating a good income - whatever industry that may be in.

It was like telling a child Santa wasn't real. I knew that I did not have the same long-term goal anymore as I saw things very differently and felt I had achieved what I set out to do already. If I wasn't a model, who was I? Who is 'Anja'?

After a few more weeks of socialising and doing more modelling, I had to take new digitals for my agency in the Netherlands. These photos were pretty dreadful, as it was hard to get the right background and lighting - not to mention I looked very sickly without makeup on (at that time). I had to retake my measurements, sending to my agency and apologising profusely I had gained a few centimetres on my hips. I admitted to them there was really nothing I could do, at 18 my hip bones just expanded to a womanlier shape, only extremely minimally, but it made a big difference.

This obsession on size had made me so disappointed in myself. I took simple photos of what I thought was my body in good shape, keeping them in my phone as a memory of when I realised my hips were "too big for modelling".

I was still booking loads of great work, and really enjoying it. I would have loved to go overseas on contract again, but wanting to just spend some time at home first, and save some money. I knew that I should consider a different long-term career path as I wanted to do something uplifting and expansive that was focussed on wellness, with financial stability.

By late August, Mum had sold our apartment near the city, and we were going to live up the coast with my father. It was strange moving back in with Dad, as the last time I had lived in that house full time was when I was 7 years old before my parents separated.

I was enjoying life up at the coast – climbing Mt Coolum regularly, starting a new vegan diet, being active, painting and connecting with nature. I was living closer to Alex, so I could spend more time with her too.

What led me to veganism was I could feel my health slowly plummeting once again and was willing to give anything a try to help my body. I knew lots of vegans get a bad rap for being pushy with their beliefs and animal activism, so when people would roll their eyes and ask if I was doing it for the animals, I would defend myself, "no of course not." I did love animals; however, my decision was health oriented.

Veganism is great, but it is hard!! I was finding it a challenge to be vegan when those around me were enjoying juicy, tasty meat, melted cheese, scrambled eggs or even just mayonnaise!

Each meal, I'd cook something authentically vegan that I just made up in my head. My diet was purely a lot of vegetables and chickpeas, hummus, coconut yogurt and acai bowls. It may just be my cooking, but nothing had any flavour.

Even little vegan treats I would get and cook wouldn't taste like anything. "Just melt some cheese on it, or have it with some aioli," Mum would say sympathetically. I think my blood sugar levels must have been low as I could almost cry when I remembered these add-ons weren't vegan and I couldn't eat them.

I could feel instability in my health so was treating my body particularly well. I hadn't been drinking alcohol as I really did not see a point, feeling as if I did not have to be drunk to have fun. Even though money wasn't flying out for nightlife, I knew that I was eating into my life savings just going to the organic shop and had to start making a good income.

After doing some research, I decided to refocus back to modelling, making connections and arrangements for October. It was to be the premier Fashion Month event to try and create a great fashion industry in Queensland by showcasing and uniting designers and Queensland talent. I was offered a job managing and coordinating the Pop-up Store with at least three days working there a week, if not more. The job evolved to be more of a constant person there and in-house model than a manager, however was volunteer.

It was quickly approaching October and I had the month fully booked.

It was going to be an incredibly busy month, made even more difficult by the fact most of these things were in Brisbane, and I no longer had a place there. Mum was commuting most days, and other times staying with family and friends. Very generously Jasmine had invited me to stay at her house whenever I needed throughout the month, so it made things a lot easier.

I started in the pop-up shop early at the beginning of October, getting to meet two designers that were down from Townsville, who were showcasing their designs in the store. I had a great time interacting with them as well as the local Brisbane designers, trying garments on almost every moment of the day and getting great photos for the event's social media, the designers and myself. If I wasn't in the store, I was off doing something else related to modelling and my career in fashion.

I had started drinking almond milk lattes and was *still* sticking to my vegan diet. One, if not both of these things were having a bad reaction in my stomach, and I could not keep food in me. This made working at the store challenging at times, as I could be the only one there in some instances and be unable to get to the bathroom. When I did have to go to the bathroom, I had to go down the escalators and across the food courts. If it was urgent, I would have a problem.

I started to stop eating altogether unless I could be near the home toilet for the following few hours afterwards. I began drinking activated charcoal smoothies as they are supposed to detox as well as slow your bowel down, and I was just needing some relief. I was expected to be in nude G-strings all day, so I could try on the clothes in the store, so there wasn't the option of wearing a pad for protection most times.

By mid-October I started teaching in a high school for a week as part of their home economics program. They would showcase their designs in a runway that I was coming to choreograph and teach the students how to do a 'fashion catwalk walk'. I hadn't *really* planned lessons out and was very unsure of how to teach 40 kids at the same time.

When I got there, I had to be given a microphone to be heard and I was standing outside with the students in the hot sun, as that was the only space big enough for our rehearsals. Things were going well, and they were beginning to listen to me and wanting to take pictures with me after class.

During the lesson on that first day, I was standing still for too long again. I began getting the black spots over my eyes, until I had to hang onto a pole to guide myself to the ground - trying to regain my sight and hearing. It was so embarrassing for this to happen in my first class.

The second day I was *so* anxious about blacking out again and narrowly escaped it. I didn't know what was going on with my body or how to control it. That afternoon I was going to get a spray tan for one of the runways I was doing on Saturday. I slept with the tan on that night.

In the morning I was lying in bed waking up, happy that I had been able to keep in the little bit of dinner I had the night before. Suddenly my stomach jolted, and I got up to run to the bathroom. By the time I had got to the bathroom it was too late. It had started running down my legs, corroding all the spray tan there. I got myself cleaned up and washed off the rest of the tan, praying that I did not have white lines down my inner thighs. What was going on with my body?

I called the school, sending my hugest apologies for having to withdraw due to illness, and asked one of the other models in my agency who is a great runway trainer, to fill in my place. I headed off straight to the doctors who was unable to give me a reasonable explanation for my black outs, and also told me the only way I could guarantee I didn't have an accident on the runway on Saturday, was to just stop eating.

I went into the runway after a three day fast and was running purely off Powerade and nothing more. The only positive of the situation was that my stomach had flattened out, completely empty.

The runway was great, but a very long day - with a 9am call time ending again at 11:30pm.

I only began eating again after a few more days as every time I tried, I had an accident from no control. I was still busy with the pop-up shop but needed to take three days off - one to prepare for the next big runway, a day for fittings and the day of the show.

I got through the fittings fine, only snacking on some brown rice and not much more. My tummy felt stable, so I was looking forward to the show the following day.

On show day, I was prepared for another 12-hour day. A few hours before the show started we were given ham and salad rolls as a light meal. My stomach was gurgling at it, but I trusted it would be okay - I had been about 12 hours without an accident. We began getting dressed for the first look, I had my own rack with more than 10 outfits, some of which were incredible international designers.

I was walking for a huge Australian retailer first. I was so thrilled to walk for this brand as it had been another goal of mine. I walked the runway confidently. As I was walking along the stage behind the curtain to line up for the finale I felt something wet drop down onto my legs. I thought it could be a drop of water from the air-conditioning as I couldn't see anything in the dark and couldn't feel anything else to suggest otherwise. I touched it with my finger and discretely brought it up to my nose and sniffed, trying to work out what it was.

There couldn't have been a worse time for my bowel to go. I shouldn't have eaten a sandwich roll. I excused myself saying I was sick, running down to the bathroom and squeezing past the male models waiting just outside the toilet. I dashed in, conscious of not making any suspicious noises. I had to take my nude G-string off and throw it in the bin. I was still in shock I could not feel anything until it touched my leg – even though it had been that way since I was reconstructed.

I tried to get my stomach under control before running back up the stairs to my rack. I was due to be walking out onto the runway in swimwear in less than one minute. I was so nervous in this moment, putting on a new nude G-string with some very small and cheeky swimwear over the top. If I had another accident, there was nothing there to hide it, and it would go on the clothing. I had to make the flash decision on whether or not to continue.

I had been working so hard for this and people were relying on me, so I went out on stage. Walking one foot in front of the other, confidently. I knew that if something happened, I was unlikely to even feel it.

After walking for another swimwear section, casual wear in short shorts and another two dresses, it happened again. I ran down to the bathroom, even more crowded by male models and had to throw that G-string away too. I hoped that I had kept another pair of underwear just in case.

I went back up to my rack, my stomach like a washing machine and my heart racing. I just knew I could not get back on that runway again this show. My poor mother and father were in the audience, waiting for me to come out again, as I said my apologies backstage, leaving the show and texting mum to let her know.

This experience could have very easily put me off ever walking on to a runway again.

I dusted myself off and got back on the happy horse. I continued with my shoots, and attended the afterparty for fashion month, dressed by an American designer who I had shot with for a magazine cover earlier in the day.

The next month began by shooting another cover for the following April before I was flown up to Townsville, courtesy of designers, to get some amazing shots of their clothes and be at their new store opening party.

It was such an exciting opportunity, and I was staying up there for four days at one of the designers' houses.

Each day was filled with millions of photos being taken in clothes made by all five designers at their collective store in the shopping centre. I loved all these designs, being around so many energetic and appreciative people and being in front of the camera.

One of the highlights, was heading out to Magnetic Island where we did a big hike up to the forts with insane 360-degree views of all the boulders, mountains and crystal clear, bright aqua ocean.

I was wearing a pair of the designer's bright activewear leggings that was designed off a silk painting she had done. They were colourful, and I paired them with an Australian outback style hat and bright bikini top. I was very brown, tanned to a healthy colour. The pictures were worth the walk, and the experience itself has made a very fond memory.

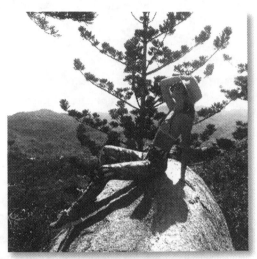

On Magnetic island

I was fortunate as by that time my stomach had settled, and I had no issues. I was able to discreetly do a wash out in the designers' bathroom late at night without any trouble.

Not long after this trip, I was off down to Sydney for a huge production runway at the Sydney Olympic Park. It was the hugest audience - a dinner with runway for a large group of people (800+) from China. It was paid well with a huge, high and long runway, fire shooting up at the edges as we walked, amazing lighting and sound production and a large group of models. I made some great friends and was incredibly pleased to have achieved another one of my goals for the year of travelling interstate to Sydney and Melbourne for modelling.

Back in Queensland, mum and I had moved back to Brisbane again, as the commute for work was getting too much. We were bunked up at one of her friends' place, sharing a room together.

As my December cover came out, I began blogging for a Queensland fashion organisation fully immersing myself in all facets of the industry. I was attending fashion events with a photographer and writing wonderful pieces to describe that event. I had never done anything like it before, but found the blog being repetitively shared and lots of people commenting on how well written it was.

After my second blogging event, I had arranged to head out into the valley with one of my good friends from high school. I hadn't been drinking at all and thought I should give the valley another chance. I wanted to have some fun and experience what all the fuss was about it.

I had a wild night out with my friend, drinking many cocktails as we danced the night away, and had handsome guys buying us free drinks. It was my first time ever being tipsy! It was one of the best nights out I have ever had, as we were just letting loose and enjoying ourselves.

Even though it was a very fun night, I had serious things to sort out… what was I going to do to get a good income?

XXIV

Learning

Understand every choice you make is the right one for you.
If you make a choice that does not produce the outcome you
were wanting it does not make it the wrong choice, it just
means you have asked to learn from the experience.

Despite making leaps and bounds in the fashion world, there was not much financial reward. Most things were paid with publicity, which is something that I cannot use to pay bills. I needed something to give me an income. I was a year out of school and thought I was overdue to pursue a career that I could do for the rest of my life.

I was encouraged by my mum's friend (landlord), my own passion and mum herself to look at other options, and perhaps get into real-estate. I did not have impressive work experience on my resume, apart from fashion, and did not have a qualification. I decided to go into the property industry as I had a love of working with people, a real-estate obsession from my parents and desire for a career that has a good financial output in relation to work input, and no glass ceiling.

My mum's friend worked closely with developers and introduced me to a real-estate agency who were interested in offering me a position in sales straight off the bat, once I got my training.

I decided to enrol to get my Sales registration and went to a week of intensive classes before getting more assignments than I could count. I knuckled down, thinking I could complete the assignments easily in a few days, however it ended up taking a few weeks as I underestimated the workload, and was doing that on top of my modelling jobs.

I was shocked when I got back a resubmit, not understanding what was wrong no matter how many times I looked at it. The wording had to be so specific, and most times plagiarised from the textbook rather than explaining it in other words.

I thought real-estate would have been a walk in the park, but it had many legal overlaps and specific systems which added a new element to it.

I had a great Christmas with my family and was planning a night out on Boxing Day. I was going to go with Jasmine and my other close friend I had the great night out with previously. I went out wanting to meet a nice guy as I had almost given up on a good one ever being out there.

We had a few glasses of rosé before going out. We were all able to hold our own, just were very giggly and flirtatious.

Arriving there, we spent a lot of time on the dance floor, and I met a nice guy who knew me from Instagram and another one I had known briefly when I was 16, Fred. I had never kissed a guy I didn't know before and wasn't comfortable with a 'kiss and run' scenario.

We were all dancing until I got tired and had to sit down while Jasmine, full of energy, danced on. I had a headache already, it felt like an instant hangover and I was just wanting some Panadol. The guy who knew me from Instagram was messaging me trying to find me, asking if I wanted to go back to his place. I just said no as I was too tired and then stopped replying for the night.

Fred's friend offered to drive my two friends and I home, and we got in the car thinking we were going to be dropped home, but we ended up at Fred's place. We all just crashed. I kept checking on Jasmine as she was not feeling well and we all ended up in the kitchen around 3:30am scavenging for food. It was a harmless night, but nothing like anything I had ever done before. I shared a few kisses with Fred and felt so comfortable and happy. I usually didn't like being touched or having people to close to me, but with him it was different. Naively, I interpreted this as a good omen.

In early January, I was almost unrecognisable to myself, and had what mum called "The weekend from hell" where I went "off the rails". I argued about this at the time but looking back I understand that mum couldn't have been more correct.

It started off harmlessly, I was heading out with one of Jasmine's good friends, that I had become friends with too over the few times that we had met. We both were just wanting a nice night out, and I had arranged to meet Fred out that night as I was intrigued by him.

Before heading out, my friend and I were in the bathroom together doing our hair and makeup, eating a nut mix and talking about what had been happening in our lives. I had bought some wine using the teenage alcohol purchasing code of buying the cheapest alcohol with the highest percentage. I was pleased with my choice of a $2.50 bottle of red wine with a 13% alcohol level. I should have known then that it must have been diluted with gasoline to be so cheap.

We both had two glasses of red wine. I did not like the taste, but I was used to drinking crap that tasted bad, like the vitamins and laxatives I would revert to throughout my life. I drank it down, as I knew people my age that could drink 10 glasses of wine without it having any effect.

When we got in the uber, we were both definitely tipsy. We had left the house quite early, around 9:30-10pm. By the time we got into the club, we decided to go straight to the dancefloor rather than getting another drink. I was surprised by the lack of control I had over my body, my muscles feeling like jelly.

"I have to go and vomit" I said to my friend - the first time these words had come out of my mouth from anything other than illness. I had no idea what was going wrong with my body, but I knew it wasn't right, and it wasn't being "drunk".

I slumped over the toilet throwing everything up. I hadn't eaten much that day, so it was all red liquid. I threw up a lot more than I had drunk, so it was hard to understand. I was drifting in and out of consciousness, and after about 40 minutes in the toilet cubicle my friend helped me out of the club to head home.

I was sitting down leaning up against one of the walls outside the club, like all the drunk mess girls I had shaken my head at just a few months before. I was having the realisation of alcohol's effect on the body.

I was drifting in and out still, and this stranger sitting next to me grabbed my friend, saying that she needed to call an ambulance. My heart was beating too fast and I could not keep conscious.

The ambulance came, and I lay down in the bed, going unconscious again on the ride to the hospital.

Next thing I knew, I woke up at 3am in the chairs in Emergency wrapped up in a blanket, asleep on my friends' shoulder.

We got in a taxi and went home. I was feeling dreadful but had a shoot first thing in the morning for one of the creative renewables designers that had flown down to Brisbane. I was up again at 6:30am to go and pick her up, and head over for the shoot. I had a bottle of water with me and was trying to stay hydrated.

The shoot went well considering my circumstances. Once I had hair and makeup on, and put on my modelling persona, you would have no idea that I was in the hospital just hours before. The images were some of the best I had ever done so I was proud of the result.

On my way home, I stopped at a friend's place, the same one I've had since I was 3. He could not stop laughing at me because he could tell I had a horrible hangover. He fed me McDonalds, we watched Sex in the City and dangled our feet in his pool.

I was so embarrassed I had missed seeing Fred the previous night due to me being taken out in an ambulance. He shot me a message that he was out for a Sunday Session and asked if I wanted to come.

I wanted to apologise for the previous night and get a chance to see him before he went back to work. I rushed home, got dressed (thank god I had my hair and makeup done already) and caught an uber out, deciding to stay sober as the thought of alcohol could not even compute through my head.

When I saw him, he wrapped his arm around me, happy to see me. I was glad I was there in his company. He insisted I have one drink at least, so I did, but that was all.

He was telling me how he had to leave as he had work early in the morning and invited me to go back to his place. I thought it would be harmless as we had such a great time last time, I thought this would be no different. I wanted to get to know him more one-on-one, and stupidly thought this was a good opportunity.

You can all already guess the story I am about to tell. We went to bed and things got heated. I had told him I was a virgin and didn't want to have sex as I wanted to wait until the right moment.

We were playing around, and he began trying to convince me to have sex. I knew that I hadn't done my dilatation in about 8 months as I had given up on the thought of having intercourse anytime soon. I told him I couldn't but wasn't persistent as I thought he would be able to tell in one second that the opening was far too small. I could feel it hurting as he tried to push in, but just relaxed as I had already told him I wasn't wanting to (not physically couldn't) have sex and thought that I would let my inability speak for me.

I couldn't be bothered sitting down with him, having the talk about the surgeries and dilatations and the short version of my life story and disability. I had been through that conversation many times, and I just wanted to be simple for a change. I was so desperately trying to have a normal teenage girl experience, as people I knew had been doing this kind of thing for years before.

I just relaxed, waiting for him to come to the realisation I couldn't physically have sex. It just hurt when he tried to push it in. A lot. It felt as if it just could not go in and was hurting around the edge, nothing more.

By the time I had realised what was happening, it was too late. My virginity was gone, I was in pain and he had finished without even putting on a condom. I was a good girl... I was not taking any contraceptives and was quite against anything that would unnaturally affect my hormones honestly.

I asked him if what I just thought happened, had actually happened. He confirmed, also trying to confirm that I was on the pill.

"I told you, I wasn't..." I said to him, still in shock. I could not comprehend what had just happened. How I could have *let* it happen. How I could not even *feel* it inside my body... the nerves really weren't there. I already knew it, but this just confirmed. I could feel NOTHING inside of me. I wanted to pour my heart out about how much effort, surgeries, pain, blood and tears had gone into this insignificant moment in his life, another tally on the board. Instead, I shut up as I did not want to scare him off.

He told me I had to take the morning after pill and telling me he could come with me to get it. I was trying to dispute it as I knew that it would make me very unwell. I didn't have knowledge of the product, more of my sensitive state of health, and how easily I could get sick from different chemicals. I told him I would take care of it, knowing fully well that I was not going to take that pill as I did not want the ramifications to follow. I thought the time of my cycle was not a window of fertility and was going to just trust in that.

The few hours to follow, I had never received so many messages from him asking if I had taken that pill.

I spoke to my best friends, a guy and a girl and they both told me to stop being stupid, I *had* to take it.

After having a shower, I did a walk of shame into the chemist to pick it up, answering all these invasive questions from the pharmacist before they handed it to me. I thought I would feel different after I had sex for the first time. Maybe it was all the propaganda that I had something taken away from me that I never got back. I felt ashamed at the position I put myself in to let it happen. I was not usually that stupid.

I took the pill, and went into mum, confessing the story to her. She was so furious, she knew how compromised my morals were in the situation and was disappointed that I had gone about things in the way I did.

"We will just have to see if you are pregnant or have an STD!" Mum said to me logically.

I went back to Jasmine's house and was curled up in a ball with severe abdominal pain and nausea. She was talking to me, consoling me. She lit some candles singing a funny song as a new start to the new year.

Within days, I was so sick. I started bleeding and then ended up in horrible pain, nausea and fevers.

I got admitted into hospital. The diagnosis was a kidney infection - the chemicals in the pill had put so much toxin into my kidney, and it was compounded by the fact anything vaginal would automatically go up through my urethra that was located in the same passage.

I was in hospital for four days. I did not receive a single message from Fred. It was clear to me that it really meant so little to him. This just made me feel more stupid about the whole situation. I could not shake this feeling of shame.

I used this time to complete my real estate assignments and submit them all.

I was trying to stay busy. I had one of Fred's friends make a move and I told him that I was involved with his best friend, and they just told me, "he wouldn't even care."

This struck a chord, and I knew there really mustn't be anything there. I wanted to stay far away from that friendship group.

I went for a job interview in real-estate, and was struck down for being a young woman, and thinking that I would be able to do well in real-estate with both my age and gender. Things weren't really going to plan anymore.

I did a few shoots, one being a great project with John that produced amazing images. This took my mind off things – my disappointment in myself, confusion at who I was anymore and stress of finding a job. I was being messaged relentlessly by people on social media, as well as guys I had met while out and made the "Fred mistake" again. I thought it would be able to eventuate into something, misjudging empty promises. By that time, I was on the pill under mum's careful instruction, and wanted to get rid of the memory of losing my virginity and see if I could feel it through being more aware and understanding what was happening.

I was desperately trying to figure out my sexuality. Despite my usual routine and sit down chat, I hadn't been open about my condition or of how greatly this intimate experience meant to me, because of all I had been through. I just wanted to do normal teenage girl things, even though it just couldn't happen. I had been through two of the same lessons, and I couldn't work it out. I wanted to understand why it didn't eventuate and blamed myself...

I also was amazed at how little I could feel inside me. The only thing I felt was pain.

One and a half weeks after this, I went for a second job interview at a real-estate agency. They liked me and said that they would like for me to start at reception and work my way up, as there were no other jobs available at that stage, and it was so busy they wanted to bring on a second receptionist.

They asked when I could start, and I said "Now."

XXV

Humility

Create a new beginning in every moment. Never hold yesterday's regrets in today's fresh start

9am the next day, I was starting my new job.

It was a sensory overload, so many new skills to learn, new regulations - working out the phone in the first place to be able to answer a call and learn people's names was a challenge. My brain was reactivating as I had a whole new responsibility and was finally earning money for myself. I was working 8:30am-5pm and began working Saturdays 8:30am-2pm as well.

In my second week there, I was noticing some strange symptoms and abdominal pain. I went to the doctor after work, only able to get into a doctor I had never seen before. I explained my symptoms to him. First, he wanted to check if I was pregnant, which I wasn't. After that, he reassessed and given my circumstances he thought I had a urinary infection that was progressing fast, so gave me antibiotics to be able to go to work the following day. I had this antibiotic hundreds of times - it was actually the same one I took prophylactically for UTIs as a child.

I called my mum on the way home as we were now housesitting an apartment in Kelvin Grove, and I was looking after their fish while the guy there was overseas. Mum was planning on commuting to the coast but after my call she thought it would be a good idea for her to stay with me that night.

I took my first antibiotics at 8pm and went to bed straight away, falling asleep instantly as I was feeling so unwell.

I woke up around 11pm, feeling like I was going to vomit. I was gagging, and mum woke up next to me asking if I was okay. I told her I needed to go and vomit, but she told me that I should be okay, and to just relax. I ran to the bathroom in the dark, leaning over the toilet vomiting out my stomach lining as I hadn't eaten.

I got back into bed, and I was telling mum that I felt so nauseous and unwell. I was beginning to whimper, and mum said I was beginning to hyperventilate and I should just relax and try and get some sleep. I woke up again not long after, vomiting again. I felt my eyes were very heavy and there was something wrong with my ears. It felt like the ear canals had turned into a hard metal rod and were going numb.

I came back to bed, telling mum again. She told me I should try and sleep as it would allow my body to heal.

Within another ten minutes I was up again. After throwing up, I told mum that I was going to the hospital, I just had to. I said mum could stay in bed and I could just drive myself and get checked out.

Mum leapt out of bed, "don't be silly, I'll take you."

We turned on the lights as I leant over the toilet throwing up. It was blood.

I looked in the mirror, my lips' size was tripled, eyes almost closed over and ears red and swollen up. My heart was racing, and I now couldn't leave the toilet, throwing up more and more blood. Mum was telling me we had to go to the hospital NOW, grabbing a bucket so I could walk and vomit.

As we got in the lift, I was leaning up against the wall. "Mum, you have to call an ambulance. Please mum. I need an ambulance". I was sliding down the wall as mum clung onto me, my eyes beginning to black out.

"Stay with me Anja, stay with me..." mum said, slapping my face to keep me awake. She told me she could get me to the hospital faster than an ambulance, completely forgetting the paramedics could resume treatment on the way.

Mum dragged me through the doors of emergency and they took me right into resuscitation. They plugged me up to machines, drips with antihistamine and fluids, anti-nausea pills and monitoring my heart. I had about 4 nurses around me and a doctor, as I continued to vomit.

They said I had anaphylaxis to the antibiotics, and I had developed that from the overexposure as a child.

By 5:30am my condition had stabilised. They sent me for an ultrasound and all looked fine. I was taken up to the ward as they had to monitor my reactions to other antibiotics, trying to find a treatment that would target the UTI without an allergy.

I was going to be kept in that day for monitoring after such a near-death experience flowing in and out of consciousness the night before.

It was awkward to call my new work, as I had only been there a week and already needed a sick day. The other receptionist was unwell as well, so that gave them the problem they were trying to avoid by hiring two.

I got back the day after coming out of hospital, blending back into work. I was still not feeling well, but desperately wanted to impress in my new job.

I was learning quickly at work, taking over the social media accounts, learning property marketing and did a lot of sales and rentals admin work. I was invited to help out at an auction, after only having been there for three weeks when at the beginning they weren't planning on letting me out into the field for the first three months. I was striving and became the only receptionist, after the other girl resigned.

I was having nice time with friends trying to balance my work life with social.

I was just focusing on work and had basically given up on meeting a good, long term partner. I really was working hard to try and get promoted within the agency faster, as the wage I was on was $13 an hour before tax, so really not enough to give me financial independence.

I had decided to share-rent an apartment with my mother as "housemates". We found a place and moved in. It wasn't glamorous, but I felt good to have a home that was half mine by financial contribution.

I had been talking to a boy I had seen out one night that had contacted me. I didn't want to engage in days or weeks of conversation only to not be able to connect well in person. I arranged to meet him out one Saturday night, after I had just worked a long six-day week.

I had been having intensified abdominal pain over the past weeks and was anxious to go to the doctor and get more antibiotics if I was becoming allergic from overexposure.

Succumbing to the pain, I went to the doctor that Friday, getting a combination of antibiotics to knock the infection on the head. I was carefully instructed to come back on Monday for review.

I started taking my antibiotics, but apart from the pain I did not feel overly unwell.

By the Saturday, I went out with two friends and met that boy at the bar. I only had one drink as I was on antibiotics and didn't want any issues. As soon as I met him, we just connected. Peter felt familiar, and as if I had known him for a long time. I felt automatically comfortable and content in his presence.

He had been chatting to me, putting in so much effort for a few weeks by this stage. I was so pleased to finally meet properly and get to know each other. I was so glad I took a chance on him, as he exceeded my expectations.

We hit it off, staying up until 2 or 3am talking.

On the Sunday I still was having bad pain, so spent the day in bed resting with a hot water bottle.

There was one bulge in the lower left area of my abdomen. It was so sensitive to touch, and even to be bumped or walk it was feeling quite agonising.

I went into work on the Monday, determined to ignore it, and ducked back to the doctors at lunch as per their careful instructions. After examining me, and taking observations, I was sent directly to Emergency at the hospital, with an urgent letter written by my GP.

I called work, having to tell them the situation as they would have to arrange someone to cover for me in reception. I couldn't tell them how long I would be there for but insisted that I would update them as soon as I knew.

I went into Emergency and bloods were taken and I was give IV antibiotics as I had clear symptoms of a pelvic infection. I was told by the doctor, the same bacteria showed up on the swab that they did in the hospital in February and I assured them that no one had ever notified me of this.

I was so upset that I had another bout of PID, as every time it is known to impact on fertility later in life. I was also annoyed that no one had told me or treated this infection having known about it for a whole month.

I called Jasmine and she came into the hospital to be with me. I was devastated and needing support. The gynaecology team sent me for an ultrasound to ensure that everything was looking okay, as it was perfectly healthy when I was in emergency in February.

The specialist gynaecology doctor came in the room, closing the curtains behind her to deliver the news. There was a 9cm x 3cm x 3.5cm abscess formed in my left fallopian tube. This could mean they would have to take my fallopian tube out, and if it had damaged anything else that would need to be removed as well.

As it was an abscess, there was risk of it bursting and spreading infection. They put me on strong IV antibiotics to try and shrink the abscess, and if it was still there they would know it is not infectious, and that they could operate.

This was at the same time as Cyclone Debbie where all the patients (maternity especially) from hospitals in North Queensland had been brought to Brisbane, meaning there were barely any beds on the ward and they were having to open extra old ward spaces.

When mum came in, she noticed that my eyes and lips had swollen up, and Jasmine agreed. I was having another antibiotics allergy. The doctors treated me with antihistamines and trialled another antibiotic giving me a similar reaction. Finally, they consulted Infectious Diseases who found one that I wasn't allergic to, as I had now been found to be allergic to three different antibiotic families.

On the second day I was surprised in hospital by Peter. I looked disgusting, matted bed hair, purple, swollen eyelids and a grey puffy face. Definitely not the perfectly made up girl he had met a few nights previous. He had a huge bouquet of white roses and some stuffed animals for me, giving me a huge hug and a kiss.

That was the moment mum decided to make a surprise entrance. I was not expecting to see either of them at the hospital at this time. Mum had no idea about who Peter was and shot me a confused look.

Saved by the bell, a doctor walked through the curtains, asking to speak with me privately. Poor confused mum, and sweet Peter went out in the hallway to get acquainted.

Lots of friends and relatives visited, bringing little gifts and flowers. I felt like a pregnant woman with my abdominal swelling, who was about to deliver her baby.

I spent the week in hospital, with Peter coming in every day, bearing magazines, food and other little surprises. He never once missed a day or came in empty handed. He would let me rest my head on his chest as we would spend the whole day in the hospital, sharing stories and making memories. He stuck by me despite the circumstances I was in. There are still good ones out there ladies.

After a few days, they did another scan to find the 'abscess' had only shrunk 2cm.

They decided to go in and operate. They explained that due to the scar tissue it would be an incredibly difficult procedure and I had to be aware of the risks. I could come out with a hysterectomy or bowel injury and colostomy if they were unable to dissect the scar tissue effectively. I had to sign away my consent, just wanting this pain to go away.

I went into theatre around 5:30pm, a week after first getting into hospital. I was really uneasy about this procedure, but I didn't have a choice. I wanted to conserve my body from the damage and pain of this 'lump'.

I was offered anti-anxiety medication through the drip as it is standard practice, however I declined, telling them that I was used to going in and out of theatre.

I felt my back press against the cold, hard, metal surgical table, sending goosebumps down my spine. The surgeons waved as they knocked me out with anaesthesia.

Waking up in recovery, I was frightened. I had a catheter in between my legs, prongs in my nostrils, blood circulation things on my calves and pain killers pumped into my veins. I felt very woozy - my abdomen ballooned swollen, and far too sensitive to touch with my hand.

"What happened? Am I okay??" I asked the nurse. She told me everything was fine, and I would have to wait for my surgeon to explain to me.

I went up to the ward, to see mum and Peter waiting there for me, just after 10pm. They were so happy to see me and told me that the surgeon had come and updated them, telling me that they had opened me up to find out that *everything* was plastered to *everything*. Scar tissue - adhesions from my abdominal wall, to my bowel, to my ureter, to my reproductive organs and this growth.

They told me that because of that I had two choices. Choice 1 - have chronic abdominal pain and the abscess might eventually 'disappear' or choice 2 - look at booking in for an incredibly complex and risky surgery to remove the abscess and separate the scar tissue that had high risks and mean I would likely to need a hysterectomy from the damage. If I was to choose choice 2, it would have to be booked in as it would be a day long surgery.

I tried to manage with choice 1, checking myself out of hospital the day after surgery, and returning back to work only 3 days after despite the recommended 2-week recovery period. I was determined it would not impact on my work. I had been posting to the work social media account every day from my hospital bed to show my dedication.

On my return to work, I was surprised with the Property Management Top Achiever award - the first time it had ever gone to a receptionist I was told. I was awarded a $100 David Jones gift voucher, certificate and the award for the month.

Peter and I became very close, and he told me he had fallen totally in love with me by mid-April. I couldn't have been happier to find someone who supported me through not only the glamorous times but struggles too.

As I was recovering, I was scared at what my stomach would look like once I took the bandages off. Even though I had three new laparoscopic scars, Peter kissed my tummy and told me I was beautiful, and I agreed that the new battle wounds were worth it for the story behind them.

It was difficult getting back into shape after surgery. Having had the muscles cut through and the uncomfortable pressure of the abscess inside me meant most exercise was difficult and painful.

I was doing more Open Homes help and was having every Saturday working until the afternoon and then weeknights and Sundays booking in shoots and fashion events when I could. I had been asked to design marketing for a new advert and did it with ease, proud to see it in one of the property magazines.

After my three-month probation, I was able to get a raise and begin being able to pay more of my bills.

Keeping a good balance, I had a shoot for a brilliant emerging designer, and after two fittings, I had the photoshoot. Everything was seeming fine, as I began shooting. I had a bit of a bubbling in my stomach so was nervous about one of the outfits - a pair of long white pants.

Without giving it thought, I carried on with my photoshoot. As I was standing still doing the profile and back shots, I began feeling dizzy again, having the black spots over my vision. I could feel my hearing cutting out, so I told them I had to stop, as I wavered to hold on to something. It was only the first look, and we had two more to go.

Throughout the shoot, my heart was racing, head spinning and blacking out time and time again, until it got to a stage where I could only be standing for a minute before needing to sit down. I didn't have a choice but to push through the shoot, despite the black dots on my vision coming over at least 5 or 6 times.

I was scared by what was happening with my body – was this going to be a new normal for me?

Luckily, I was distracted from my woes by brilliant news! A runway show I had cast for had elected me as the top model for the 175cm+ division to accompany the other top model of the 170-174cm division. I had walked for them the previous year and was thrilled to get this opportunity.

I booked in for two days annual leave, as I headed down to Byron Bay and then the Gold Coast for a two-day shoot for their upcoming magazine issue. It was a wonderful weekend as I enjoyed the shoots, loved the photos and the team of people. I was out in the rain and cold, causing my stomach to begin having issues. I was able to hold it together until I got home, however shooting lingerie with this feeling kept me a bit on edge.

I was still battling with abdominal pain and swelling. You could still feel this lump in my abdomen so clearly. It was getting more and more sensitive.

XXVI

―――――――――――――― ⸎ ――――――――――――――

Adversity

Understand there is never anything to fear, as it is only ever
your perception that makes things "scary"

A few days before my birthday I went to the doctor again about the pain, and they advised me I really had to go back to hospital.

I got up to the gynaecology ward quickly as they knew my circumstances and I was reviewed by a new surgeon. He had just come back from a laparoscopic surgery conference in USA where he was leading and teaching great surgical techniques.

When he first saw me, we went through my previous medical history. He lifted up my dress, seeing my scars and saying, "wow, you are just amazing. You have been through so, so much and you are in hospital in pain, still with a smile"

I was reminded of all I had been through before and felt comfort that I had been able to keep my spirits high throughout it.

The surgeon was very realistic and went through a process of elimination technique. He reviewed my surgical notes from April and saw that the amount of adhesions I had was unbelievable. We agreed to continue avoiding surgery until it was completely necessary. His hesitation was that the adhesions were sticking to the ureter from my left (only) kidney, bowels, this growth and my reproductive organs, binding them all in one clump to my abdominal wall.

Any dissection would be a high-risk procedure. I realised this as he ran through the possibilities; any damage to my ureter would sacrifice the kidney and then I would be looking at a transplant, or that I would come out of it with a colostomy, huge midsection scar, hysterectomy or maybe not even make it through.

The growth had been growing steadily from the last scan post antibiotics as 7cm x 3cm x 3.5cm and now it was up to 10cm x 6.8cm x 5.4cm.

They decided to try methods to ease my pain, apart from the obvious morphine being injected into my thighs and stomach every few hours. They took me down to medical imaging for a drainage, to see if they could remove any fluid from the lump.

I went in, had local anaesthetic injected deep into the sensitive area while they did an ultrasound, sticking a thick needle down to extract some of the liquid. They were only able to get an incredibly small amount out and were reassured by the biopsy that it was not malignant.

They saw in a CT scan that my bowels looked a bit compacted, and this could be putting pressure on the lump and causing discomfort. I got moved to a private room where I consumed 2L of bowel prep.

Discharged from hospital on my 19th birthday, I went home, fed up with the position I was in. It was like waiting for the ticking time bomb to explode.

I went back to work again quickly. On the Friday, three days later, my GP sent me back to the hospital. I had another scan, and the size had increased by 1cm in less than a week. The surgical team, that was now quite familiar with me, came down to see me. They said that nothing would happen over the weekend, so I could stay in hospital on painkillers, or go home if I would be more comfortable there.

Mum, Peter and I, believing in the healing properties of the sun, fresh air and ocean, decided I would go up to Dad's place and spend some time at the beach, to see if it could improve my pain somehow. I was so sick going up and down in the car, that Peter had to sit in the back, massaging and holding my shoulders during the drive.

By the Monday, I had fully lost my appetite. I was beginning to feel systemically unwell but tried to hold on as long as I could. The pain was no longer centralised but moved throughout my entire body.

I held on until Tuesday night, when the doctor sent me back to emergency. I was unable to keep any water or food down for 24 hours, my heart was having periods of racing, and then becoming dangerously slow, I was grey, had dropped a few kilograms and was in pain throughout my whole body. My abdomen was swollen up like a balloon.

Another scan showed the lump had increased to an uncanny size of 13cm x 10cm, however the surgeons were unsure of the actual measurements as it was in such an awkward position.

After my heart alarms went off every few minutes for hours, I was moved up to the ward and medicated with pain killers, anti-nausea medication and antibiotics. I was reviewed by the registrar, who I knew fondly from gynaecology clinic, and she got my new favourite surgeon to come and see me. The team decided that they had to operate on the Wednesday morning, trying to organise a day and time that it was possible. On Thursday theatre was completely booked, and they had to coordinate with other urology and colorectal surgeons to ensure they were either on call or present in theatre.

By the Thursday afternoon they confirmed that they had cleared the theatre roster in one of the theatres especially to do my surgery. They had to wait for this opportunity as using the emergency theatre would not be appropriate for a slow, long and high-risk procedure.

Friday morning, I was woken up and prepped for surgery at 5am. This surgery was serious; there was a chance that I may not make it through, or for there to be extreme damage. It was very high complexity.

At 6:30am the nurses told me that the wardies were coming up to get me. I frantically messaged mum and Peter as we were all very anxious about the surgery and they were wanting to say their goodbyes. They managed to get to my hospital bed minutes before I was taken down to the OT.

Mum held my hand as I was wheeled off, saying "see you on the other side" as she let go of my hand. Not the most sensitive choice of words mum!!

In the anaesthetists' area before being wheeled in, I let this anti-anxiety medication seep into my veins causing me to tell some really great jokes as I remember it. I told the anaesthetist that the drip I already had in kept tissuing, but he assured me it would be fine for the procedure as he was able to flush it.

I went in and was moved onto the cold, hard metal table once again. I had monitors coming off me everywhere, and my arms placed in different areas.

They were trying to knock me out with anaesthetic for minutes, with their ten second countdown not working on *this* old surgery veteran.

As my eyes fluttered to sleep, I did not know if I would ever wake up, and if I did, what state would I be in.

As I was off floating into La La land, Mum and Peter were both anxiously waiting for me, or any news. They received a call from the hospital, asking for my mother and saying that the surgeon needed to speak with her. Mum started to tear up, stressed and scared for her little girl's life. She confessed she thought it was the call to tell her about my death on the table, and she is not a dramatic about these kinds of things.

The surgeon told her that things were going well, and they could see that my ovary was engorged and black completely through, so they wanted to take that out to ensure there was no further surgery needed in the future. The ovary looked dead and rotten - probably why my body felt it had been poisoned.

Mum agreed, happy to hear the surgery was progressing well.

Waking up, I felt like I had been hit by a truck. I was in a lot of pain despite the pain killers. I had oxygen prongs in, a drain of blood coming out of my abdomen, a catheter coming out between my legs, my calves strapped up and a cannula with fluid and antibiotics, coming out of each of my feet. I shut my eyes again, unsure of what was under my sheet.

I was being pumped with pain killer as I desperately needed it. I was so weak and still fading in and out of consciousness. I was in a state where I feared I would never be able to get rid of this feeling that felt like it was a fate worse than death itself.

The doctors realised they had been giving me an antibiotic that I was mildly allergic to, as it hadn't been checked in my chart. I had thick, puffy purple eyelids from the reaction and they were searching for another treatment.

By the time I got back to the ward I had been away for 8 hours in total 1-hour prep, 5.5 hours in surgery and 1.5 hours in recovery. The doctors warned me that being under anaesthetic for such a long time would play out symptoms of a head injury for a few months before it returned to its normal state. I was glad to hear this explanation as I was finding myself frequently forgetting words, sentences and jumbling things up in my head.

I could not move, in any way, angle or direction. I was strapped up so tightly on my back and couldn't move my head much as I would get really bad spins. I kept trying to throw up from the nausea, but even gagging my surgical wounds were being ripped open again.

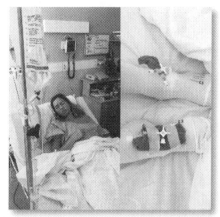

Post-surgery with cannulas in my feet

The nurses gave me laxatives as when you are having so much pain killers, by practice you give laxatives too. They hadn't realised how major the surgery was, and when they gave me the laxatives, I was unable to get up to the toilet being incontinent, and the cramps of the freshly cut intestines where they cut it away from the other organs was too much to bare.

I was told that the uterus that was bigger and may be able to carry children, was the one I just lost the ovary to. The other uterus was half the size and would be unlikely to be able to hold a baby. Not only was my fertility affected by this, but also my ability to conceive a viable pregnancy naturally.

For the first two days, I felt like I was going to die and I am not exaggerating. I was so unwell and could not move without being so ill, nor lay flat without the room spinning and the pain antagonising me. I had to have mum with me. I felt better in her presence. I was terrified as I felt like death would be easier than what I was experiencing at that time. I couldn't even lie down without everything spinning and feeling like I was floating out of my body. It gave me the most insane appreciation for just being able to wake up in the morning pain free and present - I was completely humbled and snapped out of any materialistic tendencies and the "bullshit of life" that I was caught up in before then.

I was so lucky I had no bowel or kidney injury. Coming out of surgery as well as I did, was the unlikely event, yet here I was.

My godmother and aunty came to visit me in the hospital, and I was in such a bad way physically, and also upset about the news of my ovary as I had always wanted to have my own baby. I just burst into tears when they asked me how I was. The emotion was so raw that they broke down in tears too.

I went home after four days, each day having another tube removed, learning to walk with drips in my feet and a drain in, seeing a drain removed from inside my abdomen, regaining my balance and trying to stand up straight with my pain.

I was recommended to have 6-8 weeks off work to heal properly, considering the length of the surgery and amount of dissecting they had done.

XXVII

✎

Recovery

Listen to the signs of your body always – no two bodies are the same or will respond in an identical way to any treatment or experience. You know your body better than any doctor

After three weeks in bed, I came back to work as my boss had been hinting at a promotion and I did not want to miss my golden opportunity. I was still in a lot of pain, exhausted and just holding my health together long enough to get through the day.

I was taken into my boss' office when I got back to work, and he told me that if I was selling a house or had a business lead, I would have lost the buyer or the seller. It was a good business decision that he made, but hard for me to hear. It was the nice way of him saying, "we hired a trainee for the position I was discussing with you."

I was disappointed and beating myself up. The hormone readjustment was in full swing and I was struggling to hold together my emotions.

Even when I was happy, I was breaking into tears at the drop of a hat, most mornings poor Peter would drive me into work and I would be sitting in the car crying. He had to drive me to work as I didn't get parking and would have to park and walk up big hills, and my body was not strong enough and incisions not healed. Most times I was in tears, I couldn't even understand what about. I felt like I had lost a part of my womanhood and was trying to comprehend what it would mean for the rest of my life, and if the pain would ever go away.

There were a few things that I had clarity on. Mum just had let go of one of her staff and was needing to bring another full-time person on she could trust, as Peter (now employed with mum) and the other staff member only worked part time.

I was working six days a week and my health wasn't improving - I was catching continuous viruses from other people and was finding it hard to recover from surgery with only one day relax time.

I then began to question if I wanted to jeopardise my health for a job as a real-estate receptionist, as despite the other roles I did, my job title was still just plain old "Reception". I had no idea when I would be able to get a more expansive role in the business and wanted to enhance my skills and be challenged in my role.

At that time, my mother was expanding her business further. I had always worked there on and off throughout my life, but now with a new drive, determination and set of skills, mum offered me a job. I was going to be the manager of her business and coordinate different overseas offices, business branding and development.

I knew that this would be the best option for me right then as it ticked all the boxes. New challenges, expansive role, higher income and I would have my mother as my boss who would understand when I had to go back in and out of hospital.

It was settled, I resigned from my real-estate job, taking a one-week break before beginning working for my mum, kicked off by a team bonding weekend on North Stradbroke Island.

As soon as I got into the office, I began developing and implementing systems and ensuring all legalities were in place. I project managed a major renovation of our office space, giving it an on trend, homely yet industrial feel. I began training with my mother, one of the best in the industry, learning about student counselling, visas, study options and different case studies.

Peter's birthday was coming around, so as a thank you for all he had done for me, and sticking by my side through all the struggles, I booked us a three-day trip to Melbourne with stunning accommodation.

The trip was beautiful; we get on so well when we can just be in our own bubble. We explored Melbourne, swam in the pool at the apartment, explored all the tourist destinations, shopped and ate great food.

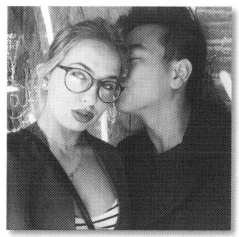

Peter and I in Hosier Lane, Melbourne

When we were in David Jones, I thought about my decision in Amsterdam to get new Michael Kors each year as a progression. I found the most stunning, versatile nude clutch with little cut out designs in it showing a metallic underlay. I bought it, funnily enough using a combination of the gift card from my real estate award and my own money. I felt so happy at this little confirmation I was back on track heading onwards and upwards.

Coming out of our little honeymoon and great moments spent together discovering a new city, we returned to work.

I was invited to go back to the high school and train runway like I had the previous October, this time with 80 students in my class. I did better than I could have ever imagined, loving teaching and directing a great show of beautiful and talented young women.

I was really enjoying taking a leadership role in all facets of my life.

My runway where I was one of the model leaders had quickly approached. I was feeling a bit uncomfortable as my stomach was very swollen and in pain once again. Because of the big surgery and not being fully recovered, I hadn't been able to do much exercise.

I ran through the motions, was shining and sweet to everyone, and had a great show. I rode again on top of that adrenaline high I got after stepping foot on a runway. I had missed it.

Mum headed off to Pakistan for two weeks in a very busy time in the office as she was hiring staff for our first offshore office. It was the ultimate test of my two months training as I resolved issues with very complex cases, and still managed to handle all emails and enquiries.

Two days after mum returned, my pelvic pain and general illness had returned, and my surgeon had booked me in for an ultrasound scan at the hospital.

I went to the hospital in the morning and had my scan. The lady scanned in 2 seconds and stopped. I asked her if she had found anything, because if she hadn't she would need to have a deeper search as I was definitely in a lot of pain.

They told me they could see a big cyst and were calling my surgeon.

Suddenly I received a call on my mobile, directly from my surgeon to tell me that I had to go down to emergency as there was a doctor waiting to admit me and I would need to be taken up to the ward and assessed for surgery.

They were concerned it may be cancerous as it did not behave normally on the scan, the matter inside could not be defined and it was 8cm inside my single remaining ovary. There was no evidence of this in the surgery I had four and a half months ago.

Much to my relief, the tumour markers came back clear. After another scan, my same amazing surgeon took me into emergency surgery at 10pm on a Friday night - organising an operating theatre, anaesthetist and bringing in people on call just for me.

I did not know what to expect from this surgery but knew my surgeon was overly capable and trusted in a positive outcome rather than the potential loss of another ovary.

I woke up and returned to the ward in the early hours of the morning. I texted mum and Peter, so they could stop freaking out, and tried to get some sleep, pushing through the pain of my third abdominal surgery in 8 months.

I was let out of hospital after two days, coming out with a fully blown up stomach and in a lot of pain. I found my pain wasn't as manageable at home, and I was throwing up for a while from the overwhelmed feeling of discomfort in my body.

My stomach was still swollen and took a while to recover with recurring sacks of fluid, bowel or something that was still palpable from the surface.

I wasn't sure if and when this would ever end. While my emotional wellbeing was improving again my physical wellbeing was in decline.

XXVIII

Finding my purpose

Understand that you attract the message you are needing to hear

It was already Christmas time, and I spent Christmas Eve with my family, bringing Peter and his younger sister along too, before flying down to Sydney on Christmas Day.

I was so unwell before my flight, as was worried I would lose bowel control from the stirring in my stomach. I was very close to cancelling my trip altogether as I did not know how I would cope.

Wanting to meet Peter's family and be with them for Christmas, I took a chance and got on the plane.

I had a great time in Sydney meeting Peter's relatives, exploring, facing the CBD boxing day shopping and visiting places of significance in Peter's childhood and his parent's relationship.

I was having severe period pain, almost at a stage where I was requiring hospital admission. The only thing worse than that, was having to get in a car with this pain and bleeding heavily, to drive from Sydney to Brisbane. I am talking about a 10 hour + drive not taking pit stops into consideration. We woke up bright and early at 4am to get in the car and hit the road before traffic.

Bless little Peter as he slept most of the way in the car. I envied him, as I found it hard to get a blink of sleep for the majority of the long drive.

I began scrolling through the posts in a Facebook group for VACTERL Association that I had recently joined. I loved reading all the posts, hearing others' experiences and having that sense that other people have walked the same journey as I have. It had only been over the past month or so, where I had been held at the mercy of my poor health that I desired to reach out to others and know their experiences. I also recalled how limiting the mothers believed the condition would be when I was in that small playgroup as a child. All of them feared how their baby would grow up, and the quality of life they would have.

Mums words rung in my head, "I would have loved to see you at this age, when you were in and out of surgeries". I knew I had to tell my story, share it even if it only uplifted one other person.

I was inspired by hearing stories of the young kids being little warriors, just like I was and yearning to comfort those mothers who feared for their child's future. I wrote a post, not even drafting it once as I was confident in the message I put out. I wrote something listing my conditions and telling them that despite it I had walked in Amsterdam Fashion week and worked as a model, and that your dreams are always possible when you believe in them, despite the condition. With this post I shared a photo of me at fashion week and then a year after, me in a hospital bed after surgery.

I posted it and put my phone down, thinking that I would get three likes and a comment "cool" from one of the mothers.

Not being able to put my phone down for long as I wasn't stimulated by much else, I picked it up again 10 minutes later. I couldn't see my background at all as my phone was flooded with friend requests, messages and comments on my post.

People were reaching out and sharing their journey as well as thanking me, telling me how inspired they were and how much me sharing had given them great hope for their child's future.

After a few days, I had at least 50 messages, 125 comments and over 300 likes on the Facebook post. I was responding and connecting with all these people. I couldn't believe there was this world of people that were so interested in how I got to where I did in my life with my birth condition. I couldn't believe how I hadn't thought logically for many years that my 'disability' was part of my story, or that there was a community that would benefit from my positive story.

I was immediately reminded of the publishing contract I got at 15, determined to write a book that could uplift the planet. I knew in that moment, that this book would be written at 19.

One of the people I connected with through my post was a man in

Melbourne called Greg who was in his early 50s. When I clicked on his profile I saw he had written a book about his condition; Imperforate Anus. After speaking with him I found he had created an Adult Imperforate Anus Facebook group and *ONE in 5000 Foundation* - a charity for those with Anorectal Malformation (ARM). It was still at grassroots level but was gaining traction quickly.

Within days of our first message exchange, we were on the phone with each other back and forth. I couldn't believe that there was another human being, regardless of age and gender, that had been through the same things as I had. I had never experienced this as an adult before.

We stayed connected, talking almost every day. We immediately became a great support for each other and shared the vision of helping the Imperforate Anus community - the A component of VACTERL.

Before I knew it, the foundation was flying me to Melbourne on the 26th of February, 2018 to be a part of the Resource and Development team (RDT) for the *ONE in 5000 Foundation* and go to the advisory board dinner with some very influential people.

Getting on the plane to Melbourne I had an overwhelming sense of excitement. I was about to meet my new "IA brother". Coincidentally, Greg was born in the same year that my late brother was. It was like having a new brother appear, who was able to understand my physical circumstances so well.

As soon as we met, conversation flowed. We had an amazing day together, meeting his mentor and co-member of the foundation for coffee. I could share my story and we all discussed the endless possibilities of the foundation.

I had the opportunity to have a consultation with the best paediatric colorectal surgeon in Melbourne. It was relieving to speak with a doctor who was so familiar with the condition, that he taught me things about myself rather than feeling like I had to educate him. The surgeon was able to give me some tips, tricks and advice, and was the first person to really explain to me the surgeries I had as a child (apart from mum!), and for me to be old enough to understand it. He told me that my surgeon who did my surgery originally was incredibly talented, as it isn't common for cloaca girls to have the urinary continence that I was blessed with.

I was counting my lucky stars as I went into the RDT meeting the following day after pondering what it would be like to meet more people who can understand the experiences of living with IA. It was a meeting with some educators and curriculum developers, as well as myself, Greg and a few mums of children with IA. It was an inspirational meeting as we established what is most important for the foundation and what the main aims were going to be. I was able to share some of my story with the mother's, and give some helpful advice as well as be a beacon of hope for their children. Both mothers had daughters that were bright, bubbly and happy despite their health struggles, and I believe that for the mums to see that this attitude can be maintained into adulthood was very comforting.

It was one of the most meaningful interactions I had with these two women, us staring deeply into each other's eyes, sharing an immediate connection and understanding as I watched their realisation that their babies can have a good life just like I've been blessed with.

I wished that meeting had never ended, I would have been content to stay in that room with that group of people forever. Blown away by the day's events, I went back to the apartment, calling Mum, Alex and Peter and sharing with them how uplifted I felt from the earlier interactions. After having a rest, I dressed in a floor length, black, backless formal dress and fumbled around doing my makeup. I was feeling confident and couldn't imagine it to be possible to be happier in that moment.

The advisory board dinner was at an authentic and trendy native Australian restaurant. We were in a private dining room with a long wooden table with black and white aboriginal art hanging from the walls. In each seat was someone who was crucial to the development and further growth of the foundation - influential people from the community, a few of the educators from the earlier session, foundation directors and little old me!

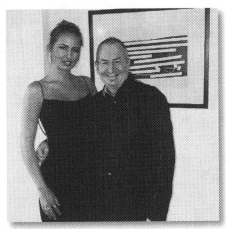

Myself and Greg Ryan – founder of ONE in 5000
Foundation and Author of *A Secret Life*

As we went around the table introducing ourselves, I was able to share my story, only to receive another very positive response. People were insisting I share my story and get some media attention. It was another confirmation that my book needed to be written, and it could not possibly come sooner.

Seeing the small difference, I had been able to make in the perspective of the mothers I had met, I knew it was the path I had been creating through every stage of my life. The different events, struggles, accomplishments and experiences built me into the perfect role model to be an impactive force on other hearts.

As soon as I touched down in Brisbane, the book writing was in full swing. Mum flew to our Pakistan office for three weeks while I took care of the onshore office. Everything running very smoothly and efficiently; I had a few more modelling jobs in my spare time and was feeling like I had found my true passion as I noted down my story on a Word document.

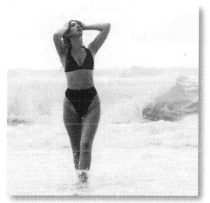

From one of my shoots at this time, photographed
by Vogue Images (David)

April came around, marking another flight to Melbourne for a RDT meeting and interview for the *ONE in 5000 Foundation*'s website. I was just as enthusiastic as the first time, meeting another mother and connecting with her, as well as meeting one of the daughters with cloaca too.

Everything was going as best as one could imagine it. I was on my way to the airport to fly home when I began having severe abdominal pain. I didn't know what it was, but it triggered the memory of the car incident in the Netherlands. I was focusing hard, asking my dead relatives for help.

When I got to the airport, I hurried to the bathroom, thinking they were bowel contractions and would go away shortly. No result. My heart was racing, and palms were sweaty. I was very dizzy as the pain was worsening. I had to try and gather myself before leaving the airport bathrooms.

When I tried to check in to my flight on the machine, it said it was no longer possible to check in as boarding had begun. I went to the service desk, asking if there was any way to get on that plane while patting tears of mascara away, smudging them on my face.

She told me I couldn't, and I explained to her my situation - how sick I felt and that I had been in the bathroom trying to get my pain under control for the last half an hour.

She immediately got her supervisor and a wheelchair. They told me they were happy to book me on the next flight free of charge, but I would need a medical certificate as a clearance to fly, as I was evidently very unwell. They arranged for me to go to the nearest doctors clinic.

I caught a taxi with a rude driver to the medical clinic while I called Greg and told him the situation. I was taken for an ECG of my racing heart which came back with no serious red flags, but my blood pressure was very high indicating a problem as my usual - sick or not - is dangerously low. My heart rate was beating so fast I was exhausted and holding my chest, I had begun vomiting and had incredible sensitivity and pain in my abdomen. I had a fever and complex medical history. The doctor sent me straight into the emergency department and said I would need review from the surgical team, and to stop eating and drinking as I may have appendicitis and require emergency surgery. I would need review from the medical doctors as well to monitor my heart and blood pressure.

I contacted Greg, and him and one of the other mothers got in the car to come and get me, taking me to the hospital and looking after me every step of the way. I was grey and feeling dreadful.

I spent the night in emergency, trying not to complain of any symptoms as I just wanted to get on a flight back home, be with Peter and Mum and doctors that knew me well and had access to my medical records.

I told them I was feeling fine, being taken to the airport in the morning by Greg's close friend and mentor and escorted to the boarding gate by him, ensuring I would be able to get on the flight. I was so grateful as my body was weak, dizzy and struggling in terms of my heart and pain level.

Within two days of being in Brisbane, I was sent by my GP into the emergency department at the hospital with concern of a bowel obstruction.

Unfortunately, this fell on Peter and my one-year anniversary. Plans were cancelled, and I was off to hospital.

They took an x-ray, seeing that I had complete loading in my large intestine. I didn't have some nerves and muscles that contract the intestine, so things would often get stuck. As I still had that bulge in my lower left abdomen, I suspected this was a pocket where there was some kind of blockage, as gynaecology had told me my bowel was very stretched by the scar tissue.

They admitted me up to the ward, organising a clean out. I had been blocked up for more than 6 months and the doctors either hadn't told me, or said I wasn't *that* blocked. I was first put in a short stay ward where I was in a room with four men, I had been given two litres of laxatives. I had no privacy or continence and would have to run across the corridor to go to the bathroom. I was so blocked that luckily, I only had to run twice.

Barely anything was coming out, and when it finally did it was clear liquid as it had just been bypassing the blockage and running out the same appearance as when I drank it. I made no progress.

The specialist I saw at clinic came to review me, prescribing 2-3 litres of bowel preparation and 6 movicol sachets a day. He explained what was in my intestines as concrete, and it would take time to flush it out. He told me they would need to get me on a new, more effective method of bowel management. For now, to get it out in theatre was too risky with my adhesions, and it was likely that would happen in conjunction with getting a colostomy.

This was the night before both my parents headed off to Denmark for my nephew's Confirmation for two and a half weeks. I was supposed to be managing the office and I was stuck in hospital trying to navigate the future of my bowels.

I was upset by this news of possible colostomy, and there being nothing else they could really do. I laid in bed visualising my bowels clear and drinking more and more laxatives. I had to be in a diaper for the amount that I was drinking, very comfortable but a little embarrassing to tell Peter.

I was visited by Peter and Jasmine in hospital and they were able to entertain me while I had my cleanout.

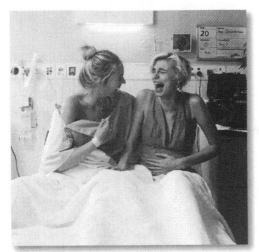

Jasmine and I, photographed by Peter - all
having a ball in my hospital room

After a few days I was taken for an x-ray. There hadn't been much progress, mainly clear liquid however the scan showed an uncanny change to my bowel – it was almost cleared. From what was coming out, nothing could explain it.

As they kept me in a few days longer, I was sitting in my hospital bed writing this exact same book you have been reading. Writing it authentically, being the unglamorous version of myself, with a smile sitting in a hospital bed, drinking a total of 12 litres of bowel prep + other laxatives.

I stayed in hospital in total a week, Greg being a great support messaging and calling me each day to check in.

I knew then and there, I had to do something to advocate and inform people about VACTERL - IA being a huge and ongoing feature of this, to give a story of hope, create a face-to-face community interaction and allow doctors to become more familiar with our condition.

From being a model, to becoming a role model. From public speaking at 11, or even standing on the dining table giving a speech at the age of three, it was all leading to this moment. Writing amazing novels at eight, and now sharing my story and condition. I can see now my past was preparing me for my future - moments that seemed insignificant then are significant stepping stones in retrospect.

My perception of my birth condition and chronic illness rollercoaster is that it is propelling me forward more than I would be without it. My desires and dreams have always been attainable, and VACTERL only added determination and appreciation for each moment. I refuse to let this illness define me, or impact on what desires I follow.

There is a large medical conference for those with Imperforate Anus/ VACTERL and similar conditions being held in America in July 2018 - an event that occurs every two years. It is an environment filled with other people going through similar things, my perfect audience. Mum had been in contact with them when I was a baby. I wanted to give back and pay it forward. I was indicated I may get an opportunity to speak to the audience and share my experiences.

Without the struggles I had been through, I would only have ever been able to express sympathy when people respond best to empathy. The reasons for the highs and lows suddenly became undeniably apparent.

In this moment, and every moment I recognise that my past does not equal my future. I believe that in the present I have the power to choose how I feel, and in what direction I want to go. From running along the path of self-discovery, I know now that my only life's purpose is to live and be happy. I now feel brave enough to follow my joy and to live it.

I pressed confirm on my flight ticket to USA. I felt alive.

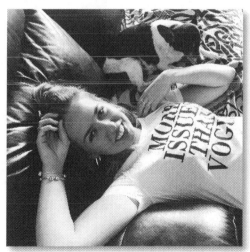

A proud VACTERL girl who isn't afraid to admit
she has *More Issues than VOGUE*

Epilogue

I thought I was living my dream on the catwalk, but I was only living a portion of it. My story is far from over; it is only just the beginning. By the time you read this, I will have turned 20 years old and be living the full version of my dream.

It will be a dream that involves connecting with you, my reader. The one who has picked up the book and has read it cover to cover. It will be a dream where I am connected globally to those affected by rare disease, in particular VACTERL and its associated conditions. No one should have to fear the unknown of the future. No one should be thinking there is no hope for their son, daughter, relative, friend, partner or even themselves.

While it is never guaranteed what the future holds for each of us, there is one thing I can guarantee...

We are the ones in control of perceiving it - making the choice to be happy, resilient and strong; or choosing that the condition is an injustice and wallowing in the pain and suffering. Both are easy.

How we are feeling emotionally determines the quality of our future just as much, if not more, than how we are feeling physically. I have had the healthiest times with the worst of attitudes and can promise I *felt* better laying in a hospital bed with excruciating pain while laughing at a joke made by a loved one.

Take a deep breath and be fearless in your declaration to be happy. Trust that all good things are coming your way. If you are facing a tough time, know that it is a sign you are strong, as you are never given a battle you cannot win, or a situation you cannot handle.

I look forward to meeting you soon X